ETHICAL DILEMMAS AND NURSING PRACTICE

ETHICAL DILEMMAS AND NURSING PRACTICE

Anne J. Davis, R.N., Ph.D.
University of California, San Francisco

Mila A. Aroskar, R.N., Ed.D.
State University of New York at Buffalo

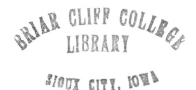

 Appleton-Century-Crofts/New York

Prentice-Hall International, Inc., London
Prentice-Hall of Australia, Pty. Ltd., Sydney
Prentice-Hall of India Private Limited, New Delhi
Prentice-Hall of Japan, Inc., Tokyo
Prentice-Hall of Southeast Asia (Pte.) Ltd., Singapore
Whitehall Books Ltd., Wellington, New Zealand

Library of Congress
Catalog Card Number: 78–51072

Designer: Karin Batten

PRINTED IN THE UNITED STATES OF AMERICA

0–8385–2273–4

RT
85
.D33

CONTENTS

PREFACE

The ethical dilemmas confronting health professionals have such broad relevance and complex ramifications that they tend to be perennially present. Health professionals have always had to make ethical decisions regarding patient care; however, our era differs from the past in several important ways. Not only do we have more factual knowledge but we also have developed technology which gives us the mechanisms to implement this knowledge. The combination of knowledge and technology has led to increased power over human lives and minds. Importantly, the rapidity in the development of new knowledge and technology makes apparent the relative nature of what we consider ordinary or extraordinary health care measures. Very quickly penicillin and pacemakers ceased to be considered extraordinary measures, to give but two examples of knowledge and technology which we now take for granted. These rapid developments have made ethical issues in the health sciences more difficult to cope with, more relevant, and more urgent. As science has provided the tools enabling us greater mastery over life and death, we, both health professionals and the general public, have raised questions which, while going beyond the issues of life and death per se, are intricately woven into their fabric. The mass media reflects these concerns in the use of such phrases as "quality of life", "heroic measures", "right to die", "right to life", and "the rights of people to humane and enlightened health care".

Although the nursing literature has dealt with ethical issues historically, a cursory glance at these works reveals that the primary concern has not been with moral principles and ethical dilemmas but rather with legal aspects and what might more properly be called the etiquette of the profession. One recent exception to this general situation can be found in the May 1977 issue of the *American Journal of Nursing.* Additionally, the American Nurses' Association has developed a Code of Ethics and the International Council of Nurses, with headquarters in Geneva, has published a book on ethical problems which confront individual nurses.*

*International Council of Nurses: The Nurse's Dilemma: Ethical Conflicts in Nursing. New York, American Journal of Nursing Co., 1977

This book attempts to bring ethics more into the mainstream of nursing education and nursing practice. All nurses face ethical dilemmas regardless of their job description and practice setting. Importantly, as the nursing role continues to change in both acute and ambulatory patient care settings and the expanded nursing role encompasses new functions and new responsibilities, nurses will increasingly face ethical dilemmas in their professional decision making.

The format which follows presents a definition and overview of that branch of ethics specific to the health sciences, called health care ethics or biomedical ethics, and draws implications for the nursing role. A general discussion of the concept, ethical dilemma, and some traditional ethical approaches precedes a more specific discussion of professional ethics and institutional constraints in nursing practice. The remainder of the book deals with the selected ethical issues of patients' rights and obligations, informed consent, abortion, dying and death, behavior control, and mental retardation. Chapter 10 examines ethical dilemmas which arise in the area of public policy and health care delivery and Chapter 11 gives examples of ethical dilemmas in specific case studies.

If, in reading this book, nurses become more aware of ethical dilemmas in health science and in nursing practice we will have accomplished our goal. We do not presume to indicate what is the right thinking or what actions should be taken in ethical dilemmas, but we do agree with Alfred North Whitehead, who said "The simple-minded use of the notions of 'right or wrong' is one of the chief obstacles to the progress of understanding".

A. J. D.
M. A. A.

ACKNOWLEDGMENTS

Although our interest in ethical dilemmas in health care predated our Kennedy Fellowships at Harvard University, it has been in this year that we have been able to focus on the complexity of these issues with little distraction from all the usual and diverse academic/professional demands and to use the rich resources in the Boston area. Therefore, we thank those who made this stimulating year possible. We wish to acknowledge our respective universities for granting us leaves and to indicate our deep indebtedness to the Joseph P. Kennedy, Jr. Foundation for awarding the Fellowships in Medical Ethics. Without the Kennedy Fellowships, this year simply would not have been possible. We hope that this book will in some small measure repay their generosity. We wish to thank all the people at Harvard who gave of their time to make this such a valuable year and we particularly wish to thank Professor William Curran of the Kennedy Interfaculty Program in Medical Ethics for lending support to this project and for sharing his ideas with us. We also thank Mrs. Najla Salhaney for the assistance she has provided and Mrs. Rebecca Ankener for typing this manuscript. And finally we wish to acknowledge that it has been our patients, colleagues, and students over the years who have given us added insights into the human condition in which all ethical dilemmas are grounded. We dedicate this book to them.

A. J. D.
M. A. A.

ETHICAL DILEMMAS AND NURSING PRACTICE

1

HEALTH CARE
ETHICS AND
ETHICAL DILEMMAS

ETHICS

Traditionally, philosophy as a body of knowledge has asked and attempted to answer, in a formal and disciplined manner, the great questions of life that any of us might raise with ourselves in our more reflective moments. The branch of philosophy called *ethics,* also referred to as *moral philosophy,* deals with important questions of human conduct that have great relevance to us as individuals and as health professionals. Ethics, as a body of knowledge, has evolved in the Western world since the Golden Age of Greece and deals with the concept of morality and with moral problems and judgments. Meta-ethics delineates the extent to which moral judgments are reasonable or otherwise justifiable, whereas normative ethics raises the question as to what is right or what ought to be done in a situation that calls for a moral decision.

The word "ethics," derived from the Greek term *ethos,* originally meant customs, habitual usages, conduct, and character, and the word "morals," derived from the Latin *mores,* means customs or habit. Today in the widest sense, these two words refer to conduct, character, and motives involved in moral acts and include the notion of approval or disapproval of a given con-

1

duct, character, or motive that we describe by such words as good, desirable, right, and worthy, or conversely by bad, undesirable, wrong, evil, and unworthy. Often, when we speak of the ethics or morals of an individual or group, we refer to a set of rules or body of principles. Each society, religion, and professional group has its principles or standards of conduct and as persons concerned with being reasonable in our conduct we rely on these standards for guidance. Not to seek guidance from such principles or rules would mean that most likely we would engage in unpredictable behavior and therefore would be considered unreliable so that others could not count on us in daily social interaction.

In discussions on this topic, the word "ethics" often becomes synonymous with "morality." Morality has been defined as a social enterprise and not just an invention or discovery of the individual for his own guidance. This social nature of morality is not limited to its being a system governing the relations of one person to others or one's code of action with respect to others. Obviously, morality is social in this sense but also, and importantly, morality is social in its origins, sanctions, and functions, since we are born into a society that has developed, and continues to maintain, mores, laws, and ethical codes.[1] As a social system of regulations, morality shares some similarities with both the law and social convention or etiquette. Convention, as we usually define it, has to do with considerations of taste, appearance, and convenience, and does not deal with matters of crucial social importance. Convention and morality share similarities in that neither is created or changed by a deliberate judicial, legislative, or executive act; therefore physical force or the threat of it does not serve as a sanction. Verbal signs of approval or disapproval, praise or blame, become social sanctions in these instances. In its focus on crucial matters of social importance, such as individual and group rights and obligations, morality shares similarities with the law.[2]

Although a standard of conduct serves to guide our individual and societal morality, we can still face ethical dilemmas. We may be ethical to the extent that our behavior elicits approval and respect from others, however, we still confront moral perplexity and moral doubt. For example, in a situation where our ethical code guides us to tell the truth, we decide to withhold truthful information because we believe such knowledge will cause psychologic harm to the individual hearing it. Such a situation confronts health professionals, particularly in caring for the terminally ill patient. This example shows that in honoring one moral principle we can violate another. In this case, if we tell the truth we may risk doing harm to the hearer. On the other hand, if we do not tell the truth, we violate the individual's right to knowledge that affects his self-determination. As one ethicist has said, the degree of confidence a community can have in its health professionals remains one critical consideration in the issue of truth telling or veracity in the health sciences.[3]

Although a set of rules is vital to human conduct, it cannot be wholly depended upon for guidance since it can never be complete enough to anticipate all possible occasions involving moral decisions. To be useful at all, moral principles must be general in nature but this also makes their utility inescapably limited.

Socrates, the patron saint of moral philosophy, in the Crito dialogue argues that we must let reason determine our ethical decisions rather than emotion.[4] In order to accomplish this we must have factual information regarding the situation and keep our minds clear as we deliberate the issue. It is not enough to appeal to what people generally think since they may be wrong, but we must find an answer by informed reasoning that we regard as correct. And importantly, according to Socrates, we ought never do what is morally wrong. The proposal as to what we should do in a situation must be viewed as to its rightness or wrongness concluded after informed reasoning and not as to what will happen to us as a consequence, or what others will think of us, or how we feel about the situation. In his arguments Socrates appealed to a general moral rule or principle that, after reflection, he accepted as valid and applicable to particular situations. But in addition, Socrates, aware of the fact that sometimes two or more moral rules apply to the same case but do not lead to the same conclusion, resolved this conflict by determining which rules take precedence over others. Here he goes beyond simply appealing to rules since they conflict with one another and establishes what he calls basic rules and derivative rules, which rest on the more basic ones. A reasoning process that establishes basic ethical rules leads to the inevitable question of how ethical principles and judgments are to be justified. A full-fledged discussion in moral philosophy develops when we pass beyond the stage in which we are directed only by traditional rules of conduct, which have limited application to complex ethical situations, and move to a stage where we think critically about an ethical dilemma in ways that allow us to use traditional rules as general principles coupled with ethical reasoning going beyond these traditional rules.

As has been indicated, not all ethical dilemmas can be resolved by an appeal to our common moral rules, and this fact lies at the center of moral philosophy as a field of inquiry. Let it be stressed, however, that the traditional interest in ethics as a subject matter must not be confused with the practical interest of moral beings. To avoid the mistake of supposing that a knowledge of moral theory is sufficient for the improvement of our moral practice, we must realize that the theoretical interest is concerned with knowing and the practical interest with doing.[5] A moralist engages in reflection and discussion about what is morally right or wrong, good or evil. A moral philosopher thinks and writes about the ways in which moral terms like "right" or "good" are used by moralists when they deliver their moral judgments.[6] If one's object is to discover unambiguous answers to ethical dilemmas quickly and effortlessly, then most likely he will be bewildered by the complexity of these dilemmas. Furthermore, he will most surely experience disappointment if he expects instant truth for one does not mine ethical dilemmas as easily as one mines diamonds, but a concern for ethical principles may prove to be the more valuable of the two endeavors.

HEALTH CARE ETHICS

Building on accumulated knowledge, especially from the seventeenth through the nineteenth centuries, advances in medical science and technology have progressed triumphantly during the twentieth century. In the wake of this progress, two sets of major problems related to optimal health care have arisen. The first set of problems revolves around the adequate distribution and availability of health care and the second set around the danger of becoming so infatuated with the technologic dimensions of health care that we cease to question their limitations. More specifically, this means that we can unintentionally lose sight of the axiomatic foundation of health care, which is that human beings cannot be understood only in mechanistic terms. This often prevalent, but limited, view has the seeds of unintentionally violating this foundation.[7] The so-called Natural Death Act in California addresses, in part, some of the issues at stake here.[8]

The health sciences make many demands upon the abilities, special training, and character of its practitioners. One of the most basic of these demands requires that we be guided by moral considerations. Health care ethics, also called medical ethics, biomedical ethics, and bioethics, is normative ethics specific to the health sciences in that it raises the question as to what is right or what ought to be done in a health science situation that calls for a moral decision. Such situations range from moral decisions in the clinical setting focused on one patient and his family to those concerned with policy decisions regarding distribution of resources. It has been argued that moral considerations in the health sciences do not differ from normal, everyday moral considerations in that both work with the same moral rules and ethical reasoning. In health care ethics the difference comes only in the special situations and issues confronting the practitioner. The task of health care ethics therefore is neither to discover some new moral principles on which to build a theoretical ethical system nor to evolve new approaches to ethical reasoning, but to prepare the ground for the application of the established general moral rules.[9] As with general ethics, we cannot expect an automatic deductive procedure in health care ethics for arriving at "the" ethical answer nor can we legitimately expect ethics as a discipline to motivate those of us in the health sciences to be moral or to reprimand us when we are not. Health care ethics does not promote a particular moral lifestyle nor does it campaign for particular life values. Its role has been defined as functioning (1) to sensitize or raise the consciousness of health professionals (and the lay public) concerning ethical issues found in health care setting and policies and (2) to structure the issues so that ethically relevant threads of complex situations can be drawn out. Health care ethics can illuminate the variety of conflicting ethical principles involved in a particular situation and can isolate pivotal concepts needing definition, clarification, or defense.[10]

HEALTH CARE ETHICS AND THE LAW

Because we use the term *right* in a very broad and indiscriminate way, the law can be helpful in giving us clues toward limiting this term to a workable definition and therefore to a more appropriate meaning. It seems certain that even those who use the word and the concept *right* in its broadest sense think of *duty* as the invariable correlation. A legal obligation is that which one ought or ought not to do. *Duty* and *right* become correlative terms and a duty is violated when a right is invaded.

In health care ethics, situations involving rights and duties at times have reached the court. Two examples can illuminate these concepts, right and duty, as dealt with by the legal system. In the case *Canterbury* v. *Spence*,[11] the patient underwent a laminectomy and within 24 hours after surgery fell while unattended and developed paralysis. The legal issues revolved around three factors: (a) informed consent, (b) negligence on the part of the physician performing the surgery, and (c) negligence on the part of the hospital in leaving the patient unattended while voiding immediately postoperatively. In examining only the first factor, the concept of informed consent is based on the belief that an individual has the right to be informed regarding possible risks and benefits of a given procedure as well as alternatives to the procedure, including the alternative of no treatment, and their potential outcomes. Only by being fully informed can the patient truly consent to a procedure since consent grounded in ignorance violates the individual's right to self-determination. One legal question in *Canterbury* v. *Spence* focused on whether a one percent possibility of paralysis resulting from laminectomy, as documented in the literature, constituted peril of sufficient magnitude to bring a disclosure duty into play. In other words, had the physician violated the patient's right to know risks and benefits of the surgery by not performing his duty to disclose this information?

Another legal case, that of *Wyatt* v. *Stickney,* dealt with the right to treatment.[12] Most of the patients, including Mr. Wyatt, at the state mental hospital in Alabama where Dr. Stickney functioned as Commissioner of Mental Health had been involuntarily committed through noncriminal procedures. The lawyers argued that when patients are so committed for treatment purposes they then unquestionably have a constitutional right to receive such individual treatment as will give each of them a realistic opportunity to be cured or to improve his or her mental condition. The argument continued that to deprive any citizen of his or her liberty upon the altruistic theory that the confinement is for humane, therapeutic reasons and then fail to provide adequate treatment violates the very fundamentals of due process. This case and the previously discussed one reflect the legal ramifications of ethical situations. Legislation and such documents as the Constitution with its Bill of Rights serve to bridge the ethical concepts of a society with its legal system when ethical dilemmas must be solved in the courts.

ETHICAL DILEMMAS

As indicated earlier, one of the major difficulties in ethical discourses is that no definite, clear-cut answer exists for all ethical dilemmas. For that reason, critical reflection becomes necessary in any attempt to deal with an ethical dilemma. Not all dilemmas in life are ethical in nature, but an ethical dilemma does arise when moral claims conflict with one another. A dilemma can be defined as (1) a difficult problem seemingly incapable of a satisfactory solution, or (2) a choice or a situation involving choice between equally unsatisfactory alternatives. Ethical dilemmas present problems or conflicts that give rise to such questions as, What ought I to do? What is the right thing to do? What harm and benefit result from this decision or action? For example, in a situation where moral claims conflict, what one considers "good" may not necessarily be "right." This reveals a conflict between two moral claims, virtue and duty. Euthanasia by some may be considered good (a virtue) in a particular situation, but not considered right (a duty). Another less dramatic example, but one that may occur more often, arises between the patient's right to autonomy and the health professional's interference with and limitation of that right in the name of health. In this instance the violation of patient autonomy becomes justified by a decision to withhold information because it is considered to be in the best interest of the patient. What is important to note here is that another determines the best interest of the patient and not the patient himself after discussing the situation with appropriate health professionals. This behavior on the part of health professionals has been referred to by some as paternalism, where the health professional's behavior reduces the adult patient or the parents of the young patient to something less than decision making, autonomous individuals.

Another example of conflicting moral claims arose in the case where a hospital superintendent applied to the court for an order authorizing the administration of a blood transfusion. The court held that the adult patient had a right on religious grounds to refuse a blood transfusion even if medical opinion were to the effect that the patient's decision not to accept blood amounted to the patient taking his own life. The court determined that the patient had been mentally competent at all times when being presented with the decision that he had to make and also when he made the decision. The court then concluded that the individual patient, the subject of a medical decision, must have the final say and that this must necessarily be so in a system of government that gives the greatest possible protection to the individual in the furtherance of his own desire.[13] The court in this case dealt with a conflict between the patient's right to refuse treatment and the doctor's duty to give treatment based on his medical judgment.

In the New York Hospital patient's bill of rights, one section, "Your Right to Decline Treatment," also addresses this ethical dilemma. It makes the point that patients do have the right to decline treatment, but also says that if the hospital staff believes that a patient's decision to decline treatment is seriously inconsistent with its ability to provide the patient with adequate care then the patient may be requested to make arrangements elsewhere.[14] This clearly draws the ethical dilemma between the patient's right to refuse treatment and the hospital staff's duty to provide treatment.

Yet another example of ethical dilemma can be found in the clinical research situation. For the purposes of discussion, let us say that a clinical researcher has developed what appears to be an effective therapeutic technique and he wishes to test its efficacy among hospital patients who have the disease this technique is designed to cure. For comparative purposes he divided the patients into two groups by random assignment so that the experimental group will receive the new technique and the control group will receive the currently accepted therapy. After a period of time elapses, the researcher discovers that one group seems to be recovering more rapidly than the other. Regardless of which group recovers faster, an ethical dilemma has been created between the obligations, on the one hand, of the scientist to complete the experiment in order to add to knowledge that can help patients in the future and, on the other hand, the obligation of the clinician to provide the present patients with the most effective treatment available.[15]

The concept of health care as a right rather than a privilege has gained broad acceptance among consumer groups although segments of the medical profession oppose this view. In the arena of public policy, attempts continue in making this philosophical stance fit with the realities of health care delivery. The preamble to the World Health Organization Constitution says that the enjoyment of the highest attainable standard of health is one of the fundamental rights of every human being without distinction of race, religion, political belief, economic, or social conditions.[16] In the United States at present, the vast majority of private health insurance plans are geared to the gainfully employed, with limited protection for the low-wage worker and none for the unemployed and the poor.[17] The attempt to define health care as a right rather than as a commodity available according to the personal resources of the consumer has given us Medicare and Medicaid and has been the basis for the on-going discussion regarding National Health Insurance.

Any number of ethical dilemmas will not only be discussed during the development of public policy, but will also continue even after policy becomes enacted into law. The possibility of legislating ethical dilemmas out of the health care scene seems extremely remote. Regardless of the type of health care system, ethical dilemmas will continue to confront health care providers.

PROFESSIONAL OATHS AND CODES OF ETHICS IN THE HEALTH SCIENCES

Health care ethics, concerned with rights, duties, and obligations, calls for an interdisciplinary quest for the structures of responsibility.[18] To understand the present situation, an examination of the remote and recent past as reflected in professional oaths and codes of ethics should prove fruitful. Although all health professional groups have oaths and/or codes, this discussion focuses only on medicine and nursing.

Hippocrates, born on the Island of Cos in the fifth century B.C., became well known throughout Greece as a practicing physician. His attitude toward medicine threw off the religious aspects of suffering and made a beginning toward the scientific study of disease.[19] Today we remember him best for the Hippocratic Oath that doctors take upon graduation from medical school.

THE HIPPOCRATIC OATH

I swear by Appollo Physician and Asclepius and Hygieia and Panaceia and all the gods and goddesses, making them my witnesses, that I will fulfill according to my ability and judgment this oath and this covenant:

To hold him who has taught me this art as equal to my parents and to live my life in partnership with him, and if he is in need of money to give him a share of mine, and to regard his offspring as equal to my brothers in male lineage and to teach them this art—if they desire to learn it—without fee and covenant; to give a share of precepts and oral instructions and all the other learning to my sons and to the sons of him who has instructed me and to pupils who have signed the covenant and have taken an oath according to the medical law, but to no one else.

I will apply dietetic measures for the benefit of the sick according to my ability and judgment; I will keep them from harm and injustice.

I will neither give a deadly drug to anybody if asked for it, nor will I make a suggestion to this effect. Similarly I will not give to a woman an abortive remedy. In purity and holiness I will guard my life and my art.

I will not use the knife, not even on sufferers from stone, but will withdraw in favor of such men as are engaged in this work.

Whatever houses I may visit, I will come for the benefit of the sick, remaining free of all intentional injustice, of all mischief, and in particular of sexual relations with both female and male persons, be they free or slaves.

What I may see or hear in the course of the treatment or even outside of the treatment in regard to the life of men, which on no account one must spread abroad, I will keep to myself holding such things shameful [more accurately: 'unspeakable'] to be spoken about.

If I fulfill this oath and do not violate it, may it be granted to me to enjoy life and art, being honored with fame among all men for all time to come; if I transgress it and swear falsely, may the opposite of all this be true.

Primarily a pronouncement of medical ethics, this oath is not a set of laws enforced upon the physician by an authority but rather a guide which he accepts of his own free will. Far from being a legal document, the Hippocratic Oath is a solemn promise given by the conscience of the physician who swears to it. The doctor's oath can be found in a number of variant forms such as Christian, Arabic, and Buddhist, and the Oath of Charaka used in India, and all share some similarities.[20]

The Hippocratic tradition in medicine has led Paul Ramsey to remark that no profession comes close to medicine in its concern to inculcate, transmit, and keep in constant repair its standards governing the conduct of its members.[21] The strengths of the Hippocratic tradition, a vital center of responsible medicine today, emphasize the importance of covenant fidelity between physician and student and physician and patient. Medicine, as a social contract, functions on the basis of this covenant. Again, Ramsey says that justice, fairness, righteousness, faithfulness, canons of loyalty, the sanctity of life, *hesed,* agape, or charity are some of the names given to the moral quality of attitudes and of action owed to all people by any individual who steps into a covenant with another.[22] The Hippocratic tradition also reveals several weaknesses. Both the ethical and medical conceptions are pretechnologic, so limits exist in utilizing it to probe the problems posed by technology. Additionally, the tradition's focus on crisis treatment as opposed to health promotion and maintenance, along with the model of the physician as a receptacle to whom people come, require reexamination. Nevertheless, the oath has not only survived all these centuries but because it anchors responsibility in the moral power and ability of the human being it exerts influence on the practice of medicine today.

In 1971 the Judicial Council of the American Medical Association developed ten ethical principles to serve as standards of conduct for the physician. They address the duties, obligations, and rights of the medical practitioner.

PRINCIPLES OF MEDICAL ETHICS

Preamble

These principles are intended to aid physicians individually and collectively in maintaining a high level of ethical conduct. They are not laws but standards by which a physician may determine the propriety of his conduct in his relationship with patients, with colleagues, with members of allied professions, and with the public.

Section 1

The principal objective of the medical profession is to render service to humanity with full respect for the dignity of man. Physicians should merit the confidence of patients entrusted to their care, rendering to each a full measure of service and devotion.

Section 2

Physicians should strive continually to improve medical knowledge and skill, and should make available to their patients and colleagues the benefits of their professional attainments.

Section 3

A physician should practice a method of healing founded on a scientific basis; and he should not voluntarily associate professionally with anyone who violates this principle.

Section 4

The medical profession should safeguard the public and itself against physicians deficient in moral character or professional competence. Physicians should observe all laws, uphold the dignity and honor of the profession and accept its self-imposed disciplines. They should expose, without hesitation, illegal or unethical conduct of fellow members of the profession.

Section 5

A physician may choose whom he will serve. In an emergency, however, he should render service to the best of his ability. Having undertaken the care of a patient, he may not neglect him; and unless he has been discharged he may discontinue his services only after giving adequate notice. He should not solicit patients.

Section 6

A physician should not dispose of his services under terms or conditions which tend to interfere with or impair the free and complete exercise of this medical judgment and skill or tend to cause a deterioration of the quality of medical care.

Section 7

In the practice of medicine a physician should limit the source of his professional income to medical services actually rendered by him, or under his supervision, to his patients. His fee should be commensurate with the services rendered and the patient's ability to pay. He should neither pay nor receive a commission for referral of patients. Drugs, remedies or appliances may be dispensed or supplied by the physician provided it is in the best interests of the patient.

Section 8

A physician should seek consultation upon request; in doubtful or difficult cases; or whenever it appears that the quality of medical services may be enhanced thereby.

Section 9

A physician may not reveal the confidences entrusted to him in the course of medical attendance, or the deficiencies he may observe in the character of patients, unless he is required to do so by law or unless it becomes necessary in order to protect the welfare of the individual or of the community.

Section 10

The honored ideals of the medical profession imply that the responsibilities of the physician extend not only to the individual, but also to society where these responsibilities deserve his interest and participation in activities which have the purpose of improving both the health and the well-being of the individual and the community.

In 1948 the general assembly of the World Medical Association in Geneva adopted an International Code of Medical Ethics and the Declaration of Geneva. These documents served to reaffirm the traditional professional commitments of the physician.

Nursing, before the late nineteenth century, was closely allied with religion and religious orders so its practitioners followed the ethics developed within these religious contexts. With the social change accompanying industrialization in England, nursing began to be practiced by untrained and socially marginal individuals. Florence Nightingale (1820-1910), the founder of modern nursing, became famous for her organizational and training endeavors for nurses during the Crimean War and later, in 1860, opened the Nightingale Nursing School at St. Thomas's Hospital, London. In a 1893 paper she wrote that sick persons must be treated rather than the disease, that prevention is infinitely better than cure, that universal hospitalization will not give positive health, and that nursing must hold to its ideals but must change some of its methods.[23] These ideals she referred to are reflected in a pledge which countless nurses around the world have taken.

THE FLORENCE NIGHTINGALE PLEDGE

I solemnly pledge myself before God and in presence of this assembly;

To pass my life in purity and to practice my profession faithfully.

I will abstain from whatever is deleterious and mischievous and will not take or knowingly administer any harmful drug.

I will do all in my power to maintain and elevate the standard of my profession and will hold in confidence all personal matters committed to my keeping and family affairs coming to my knowledge in the practice of my calling.

With loyalty will I endeavor to aid the physician in his work, and devote myself to the welfare of those committed to my care.

The International Council of Nurses in Geneva updated its code of ethics in 1973. This document addresses the duties, obligations, and rights which nurses have.

1973 CODE FOR NURSES

Ethical Concepts Applied to Nursing

The fundamental responsibility of the nurse is fourfold: to promote health, to prevent illness, to restore health and to alleviate suffering.

The need for nursing is universal. Inherent in nursing is respect for life, dignity and rights of man. It is unrestricted by considerations of nationality, race, creed, colour, age, sex, politics or social status.

Nurses render health services to the individual, the family and the community and coordinate their services with those of related groups.

Nurses and People

The nurse's primary responsibility is to those people who require nursing care.

The nurse, in providing care, respects the beliefs, values and customs of the individual.

The nurse holds in confidence personal information and uses judgment in sharing this information.

Nurses and Practice

The nurse carries personal responsibility for nursing practice and for maintaining competence by continual learning.

The nurse maintains the highest standards of nursing care possible within the reality of a specific situation.

The nurse uses judgment in relation to individual competence when accepting and delegating responsibilities.

The nurse when acting in a professional capacity should at all times maintain standards of personal conduct that would reflect credit upon the profession.

Nurses and Society

The nurse shares with other citizens the responsibility for initiating and supporting action to meet the health and social needs of the public.

Nurses and Co-Workers

The nurse sustains a cooperative relationship with co-workers in nursing and other fields.

The nurse takes appropriate action to safeguard the individual when his care is endangered by a co-worker or any other person.

Nurses and the Profession

The nurse plays the major role in determining and implementing desirable standards of nursing practice and nursing education.

The nurse is active in developing a core of professional knowledge.

The nurse, acting through the professional organization, participates in establishing and maintaining equitable social and economic working conditions in nursing.

In order to provide one means of professional self-regulation, the American Nurses' Association revised its Code of Ethics, which had originally been adopted in 1950. This code indicates the nursing profession's acceptance of the responsibility and trust with which it has been invested by society. The requirements of the Code may often exceed, but are not less than, those of the law. While violation of the law subjects the nurse to criminal or civil liability, the Association may reprimand, censure, suspend, or expel members from the Association for violation of the Code.

CODE FOR NURSES

1. The nurse provides services with respect for human dignity and the uniqueness of the client unrestricted by considerations of social or economic status, personal attributes, or the nature of health problems.
2. The nurse safeguards the client's right to privacy by judiciously protecting information of a confidential nature.
3. The nurse acts to safeguard the client and the public when health care and safety are affected by the incompetent, unethical, or illegal practice of any person.

4. The nurse assumes responsibility and accountability for individual nursing judgments and actions.
5. The nurse maintains competence in nursing.
6. The nurse exercises informed judgment and uses individual competence and qualifications as criteria in seeking consultation, accepting responsibilities, and delegating nursing activities to others.
7. The nurse participates in activities that contribute to the ongoing development of the profession's body of knowledge.
8. The nurse participates in the profession's efforts to implement and improve standards of nursing.
9. The nurse participates in the profession's efforts to establish and maintain conditions of employment conducive to high quality nursing care.
10. The nurse participates in the profession's effort to protect the public from misinformation and misrepresentation and to maintain the integrity of nursing.
11. The nurse collaborates with members of the health professions and other citizens in promoting community and national efforts to meet the health needs of the public.

One tradition that evolved from historical events in this century must be included in any discussion of health care ethics. The ethos of the health sciences, particularly its experimental concepts, has been profoundly influenced by the Nuremberg experience. The seeds of the Nazi medical experiments conducted during the Second World War grew in the soil of a number of historical and social trends. In the 1800s German medicine and universities participated in the insidious beginnings of anti-Semitism. A number of changes affected the physician who, no longer an individual entrepreneur, became responsible to express the values of the prevailing social order. By the 1920s emphasis on public health and preventive medicine focused on the desire to perfect the Nordic "species" by eliminating all impurities and defects.[24]

The Nazi medical research, which Shirer calls a tale of horror, included such experiments on concentration camp inmates as sterilization, being placed in pressure chambers and forced to endure high-altitude atmospheres until they died, tests on the effects of weightlessness and rapid fall, and freezing experiments in ice and snow.[25] The K-tenology, or the science of killing, led the Nazis to inject inmates with lethal doses of typhus and jaundice, to give gas, gangrene wounds, bone grafting, and direct injections of potassium and cyanide into the heart. The physicians dissected inmates alive to observe brain and heart action. And finally, at the height of sadism, the motivation for the macabre experiments was to collect different shapes of skulls and to retrieve human skin in order to make lampshades. This immolation of medical ethics on a massive scale by Nazi physicians proceeded unopposed by the German medical profession.[26] Out of this experience came the Nuremberg Code, which gives us valuable insights and directives to current research involving human subjects. One of the greatest contributions of this code is the precision with which it discusses the criterion of informed consent. The single most important ethical insight gleaned from the Nuremberg tradition is that it reminds us of the potential evil in human beings and serves to constantly refute the myth of inevitable progress.

Although not an ethical code per se, the American Hospital Association has developed a Patient's Bill of Rights which has implications for health care ethics. The patient has the right:

1. To considerate and respectful care
2. To obtain from the physician information regarding his diagnosis, treatment, and prognosis
3. To give informed consent before the start of any procedure or treatment
4. To refuse treatment to the extent permitted by law
5. To privacy concerning his own medical care program
6. To confidential communication and records
7. To expect the hospital will make reasonable response to a patient's request for service
8. To information regarding relationship of his hospital to other health and educational institutions insofar as his care is concerned
9. To refuse to participate in research projects
10. To expect reasonable continuity of care
11. To examine and question his bill
12. To know the hospital rules and regulations that apply to patients' conduct.[27]

One critic of the AHA Patient's Bill of Rights calls it a well-intended, though timid, document and objects because he believes that it perpetuates the very paternalism that precipitated the abuses. He maintains that such a document creates the impression that the hospital is granting these rights to the patient. But since these rights were vested in the patient to begin with, the hospital has no power to grant these rights. He argues that the title seems both pretentious and deceptive since if the rights have been violated they have been done so by the hospital and its staff. In effect, the document returns to the patient, with an air of largesse, some of the rights hospitals previously stole from him.[28]

Three other documents, not discussed here but that speak of the concept of human rights and that have implications for health care ethics, are the Declaration of Helsinki, the Preamble to the World Health Organization Constitution, and the United Nations International Covenant on Human Rights. Since so many factors influence health and illness, these documents, addressing the larger social, economic, cultural, civil, and political rights, provide a matrix for health care ethics.

THE ROLE OF THE ETHICIST

To the extent that we confront and attempt to deal with ethical dilemmas in health care by ethical reasoning, we are assuming the role of an ethicist. However, an individual not directly involved in the care of the patient can help by bringing his particular expertise to the situation. This person can assist to structure the ethical issues involved in any ethical dilemma and provide another perspective grounded, not so much in the health sciences, but in philosophy and theology. Some health care centers now have an ethicist on the staff to assist the physicians, nurses, and others who ultimately must resolve specific ethical dilemmas and act on the decisions made.

The issues before us have been stated clearly by Walter Mondale, then senator from Minnesota, when he introduced a bill to establish a National Advisory Commission on Health Science and Society. He said that we face an increasing number of new and far-reaching technologic possibilities that make the need for wise, deliberate, and sober decisions obvious. The impact on our ideas of free will, birth and death, and the good life is likely to be more staggering than any manipulation performed.[29] The likelihood that most, if not all, individuals in this country will be affected by these advancements increases with time. Present and future advancements will produce any number of medical miracles, but in addition will also produce increasingly more and more complex ethical dilemmas. The ethicist can play an important role in the deliberation of these complex issues. As nurses are even more affected by these situations, in the future they will need ways of thinking about ethical dilemmas so that they can participate actively in the decision and possible resolution of these dilemmas.

REFERENCES

1. Frankena WK: Ethics, 2nd ed. Englewood Cliffs, NJ, Prentice-Hall, 1973, p 6
2. Ibid, p 7

3. Bok S: Truth-telling and deception in medicine. Aaron Therman Memorial Lecture, Beth Israel Hospital, Boston, November 1976
4. Frankena WK: op cit, p 2
5. Melden AI (ed): Ethical Theories, 2nd ed. Englewood Cliffs, NJ, Prentice-hall, 1967, p 3
6. Hudson WD: Modern Moral Philosophy. Garden City, NJ, Doubleday, 1970, p 1
7. Guttentag OE: Introduction. In Babbie ER: Science and Morality in Medicine. Berkeley, University of California Press, 1970, pp ix–xii
8. California Assembly Bill No. 3060. Natural Death Act, 1976
9. Closer KD: Medical ethics: some uses, abuses, and limitations. N Engl J Med 293:384–87, 1975
10. ——: What is medical ethics? Ann Int Med 80:657–60, 1974
11. Canterbury v. Spence, 464 F (2d 772, 1972)
12. Wyatt v. Stickney, 325 F Supp 781 (M.D. Ala. 1971)
13. Erickson v. Dilgard, 252 (N.Y.S. 2d 705, 1962)
14. The New York Hospital, Your Bill of Rights. New York, 1976
15. Babbie ER: Science and Morality in Medicine. Berkeley, University of California Press, 1970, pp. 16–17
16. World Health Organization: Preamble to the Constitution of the World Health Organization. Geneva, WHO, July 1948
17. Zasowaka MAA: The philosophical index of health care delivery in our culture. In Leininger M (ed): Health Care Issues. Philadelphia, Davis, 1974, pp. 9–10
18. Vaux K: Biomedical Ethics. New York, Harper & Row, 1974, p xvi
19. Hippocrates: The Theory and Practice of Medicine. New York, Philosophical Library, 1964
20. Goodfield J: Reflections on the Hippocratic Oath. Hastings Cent Rep 1:February 1973, pp 79–92
21. Ramsey P: The Patient as Person. New Haven, Yale University Press, 1970, p xii
22. Ibid, p xiii
23. Bishop NJ, Goldie S: A Bio-Bibliography of Florence Nightingale. London, International Council of Nurses, 1962
24. Vaux: op cit, p 27
25. Shirer WL: The Rise and Fall of the Third Reich. Greenwich, Fawcett, 1960, p 1274
26. Mitscherlich A, Mielke F: Doctors of Infamy. New York, Henry Schuman, 1949, p 200
27. American Hospital Association: Patient's Bill of Rights. Chicago, 1970.
28. Gaylin W: The patient's bill of rights. Sat Rev Sci, March 1973, p 22
29. Mondale WF: The issues before us. Hastings Cent Rep, June 1971, p 1

2

ETHICAL
APPROACHES

INTRODUCTION

Ethical dilemmas in the nursing profession are nothing new. Yet the development of new technologies affects the nature and substance of these dilemmas in the interrelationships of nurses and patients as individuals and members of an increasingly complex society. Enlarged responsibilities for all health professionals is the outcome.

The nurse is concerned with values, choices and priorities related to the "good" of the individual, the profession, and the society. What is needed is a systematic way of approaching ethical issues facing nursing at all levels from the individual physician–nurse–patient encounter to the level of policy making for delivery of health and nursing care. The notion of an approach suggests a way or ways of analyzing or conceptualizing decisions and choices in the ethical dimensions of practice rather than ready-made answers. This chapter is a discussion of historical and contemporary moral positions that can be used to look at nurse-patient relationships containing ambiguities and conflicts of rights and duties. These selected theories and positions of historical and contemporary ethicists are commonly discussed in dealing with ethical dilemmas in health care. While they do not provide answers per se they do go beyond what Callahan calls ethical slogans or one-sentence general principles for justifying moral judgments and actions.[1]

The general concern of ethics has to do with what is behind the judgments we make. Moral philosophers beginning with Socrates, Plato, and Aristotle have for centuries attempted to answer the two major questions of ethics: What is the meaning of right? of good? and, What ought I to do? What is the morally right thing to do in this situation? The first question is in the area of meta-ethics; the second is in the area of normative or applied ethics as mentioned in Chapter 1. Health professionals are primarily concerned with the second question in the area of normative ethics. Normative ethics attempts to justify one form of behavior over another, to determine the right-making characteristics of action, for purposes of carrying out duties and obligations. The nurse, often in a situation vis-à-vis a patient, group, or community that requires the identification of alternative courses of action, must make a choice as to what he or she will do when there is conflict of rights and obligations between patients, families, other health workers, and the community. Selected moral positions will be discussed briefly to suggest different ways of thinking about conflicts that lead to choices for action or nonaction in patient–provider relationships.

One needs data in order to proceed with discussion of the question about the morally right thing to do in a given situation. The process of reflective thinking provides data by asking questions related to identifying the actors in the situation, the required action, possible and probable consequences of the proposed action, the intention or purpose of the action, the range of alternatives or chocies, and the context of the action. This process indicates that the methods of thinking in science and ethics are not mutually exclusive. One goes through a similar process in asking questions about the world of nature and the world of values. The data base is different.

Various ethical positions provide different ways of structuring these data, which lead to the same or different decisions for action. These approaches assume that the nurse has already identified a situation where a conflict of duties, obligations, or interests exists. The nurse seeks the "best" or "right" action to take when the alternatives seem equally undesirable, e.g., lying versus truth telling or allocation of scarce nursing manpower resources.

TRADITIONAL POSITIONS

The traditional positions or theories of egoism, deontology (formalism), and utilitarianism provide us with various ways of looking at health care dilemmas from an ethical standpoint. The "agent" referred to in this chapter for discussion purposes is the nurse.

Egoism

In the egoist position the agent answers the question about the morally right thing to do by saying that something is good because I desire it. The right act is the one that maximizes the pleasure of the agent asking the question. In considering alternatives the agent only considers his own comfort. The nurse would decide to lie to a patient or family member because it was most comfortable for one's self not considering how this decision would affect the others involved.

This approach has a variety of limitations. It says nothing about the moral struggle that confronts the agent. It certainly does not help the nurse in a specific conflict of values about a terminally ill patient and euthanasia, for example. The means may include giving benefits to others but that is not the end in view. The ethical egoist maintains that everyone should act and judge by the standard of his own advantage in terms of right and wrong. Even if one considers feelings of altruism, the egoist maintains that we may do things for others but one's own pleasure is the goal.[2]

Deontology

The deontologic or formalist approach suggests that rightness or wrongness of actions depends on more than the agent's pleasure or consequences of the proposed action. Rightness or wrongness depends on the nature or form of these actions in terms of their moral significance, e.g., keeping a promise. Moral significance is attached to certain relationships as well. For example, the parent–child or the nurse–patient relationship forms the basis for one's duties and obligations. In this tradition, there are both act-deontologists and rule-deontologists, i.e., obligations in relationships may be based on performing certain actions or adhering to certain rules or principles.

In act-deontology the moral values of the individual agent are of major significance. For example, in a given situation in the home setting, the moral values of the community health nurse would play an important part in decisions made about kinds of information given to the family. This position requires commitment to the principle of universalizeability. That is when one makes a moral judgment in a given situation, one will make the same judgment in any similar situation regardless of time, place, or persons involved. If one judges X to be right or good in this situation, then one must judge that anything like X is right or good in any similar situation.[3] In any home setting given a similar situation, the nurse would give the same kinds of information, e.g., birth control methods. According to this theory one has only rules of thumb to go by. There are no criteria, standards, or guiding principles to go by as in rule-deontology. One simply gets all the facts and makes a decision. An act is made right simply by choosing it.

Some critics of act-deontology claim that it is not helpful in terms of moral guidance because it is difficult to do without rules. One may not always have time and energy to judge each situation in and of itself.[4]

The rule-deontologist suggests there are standards for choosing, judging, and reasoning morally. The standard consists of fairly specific rules such as keeping promises and telling the truth. These rules say that we should act in a certain way in a given situation. X is the right act because I should always tell the truth or do unto others as you would have others do to you—the Golden Rule.

One problem with rule-deontology is that rules sometimes conflict and one has to decide which rule takes precedence over another. Another problem is the exception to the rule. In dealing with this problem, Ross distinguishes between actual duty and *prima facie* duty. He says that every rule of actual duty has exceptions, but *prima facie* duties have no exceptions. They are obligations that one must always try to fulfill, e.g., fidelity, gratitude, and justice.[5] But what if *prima facie* duties conflict with each other in a given situation? For example, if the nurse is spending most of her time caring for a seriously ill patient, she cannot give her attention to other patients on her unit. While caring faithfully for one patient, other patients on the unit may not be getting just or fair treatment from the nurse.

One way the rule-deontologist deals with conflict of *prima facie* duties is an appeal to the Divine Command Theory: an act is right or wrong because it is commanded or forbidden by God. This has problems for both believers and nonbelievers. If God commands cruelty and injustice, then it is obligatory to carry out a cruel or unjust act—an obvious dilemma.[6]

Immanuel Kant provides us with another way out of the problem of conflicting rules. Writing in the late eighteenth century, he states that one should "act only on that maxim which you can at the same time will to be a universal law," the major form of the categorical imperative.[7] A common example of this imperative is the mother who asks a misbehaving child, "What if everyone did what you're doing?" Another form of the categorical imperative says that persons should always be treated as ends and never as means. This can be a problem for the researcher who uses human subjects. Individuals may be seen as means to a particular research goal only.

Kant says that categorical imperatives are unconditional commands, morally necessary and obligatory under any circumstances.[8] It is one's duty to obey categorical imperatives with no exceptions. One does not look at the consequences first. Each person is autonomous, his own moral authority. One's own motives count for everything. There is no external authority to tell one what to do.[9]

Kant's position does not really help us with the resolution of specific moral conflicts. If one tries to apply the Kantian position, then is it possible to detach the idea of duty and obligations from ends, purposes, wants, and needs in a given situation? For example, if the goal is to return the institutionalized mentally retarded to the community, can one consider the specific needs of the individual mentally retarded person who now has to live in a rooming house? Can the individual health professional or researcher be independent of the given social order of which he is a part? History gives us a negative reply.[10]

In summary, the deontologic position focuses on moral significance of the values of the agent and on duties and obligations guided by specific rules and principles. This position does not help the agent resolve a situation where duties and obligations conflict. It does not resolve the dilemma for the nurse who decided to follow the rule that one should always tell the truth but realizes that the truth will undoubtedly hurt a particular patient in a given situation.

Utilitarianism

The theory of utility generally defines the "good" as happiness or pleasure and "right" as maximizing the greatest good and least amount of harm for the greatest number of persons. This position assumes that one can weigh and measure harm and benefit and come out with the greatest possible balance of good over evil. In the calculus of utility each individual counts as one.

Bentham and Mill present the major historical arguments for the position of utility as a standard against which the rightness and wrongness of actions are to be compared. This position, sometimes known as "calculus morality," calculates the effects of all alternative actions on the general welfare of present and future generations in a given situation. Some moral philosophers distinguish between rule- and act-utilitarianism. One seeks to determine acts and rules having the greatest utility in a broad sense of usefulness, pleasure, and happiness, an exceptionless rule. The agent looks at actions and rules in terms of what the consequences would be for the general welfare if everyone acted similarly in a given situation.[11] What if every hospital decided to have a renal dialysis unit? What would be the consequences for the general population that needs primary care services?

Immediately one is faced with the problem of whether this position involves the total happiness for a few or the average happiness for all. A crucial question is whether or not what one does in a particular situation contributes to the greatest general good or the least amount of harm for everyone. But how can everyone's welfare really be considered? Critics bring up several other problems. They accuse the utilitarian of ignoring the personal nature of good, e.g., in truth telling and promise keeping. All actions need not be considered in light of the overall general welfare. Individuals count. The utilitarian tradition is often invoked in making decisions about health care delivery. This is in direct conflict with the medical ethic; one does everything possible for the individual patient. Certain groups may accept benefits without making sacrifices raising the question of justice and fairness. Utility is not the only criterion in making moral judgments. Actually, if one adds the notion of distributing the good as widely as possible through society, one adds the principle of justice to the principle of utility for making ethical judgments. This is no longer pure utilitarianism. From this point of view utility by itself cannot be the only basic standard or first principle of right and wrong.[12]

To summarize, the egoistic, deontologic, and utilitarian traditions offer different perspectives from which moral judgments might be made. Each position has limitations when applied to specific ethical dilemmas in nursing and health care delivery.

CONTEMPORARY POSITIONS

Some modern philosophers offer other positions to look at ethical dilemmas and get beyond the unresolved problems one is left with in the egoistic, deontologic, and utilitarian traditions. Shades of utilitarianism and deontology may be detected in some of these newer positions.

Theory of Obligation

Frankena's theory of obligation takes two principles as basic: the principle of beneficence and the principle of justice as equal treatment. The principle of beneficence asks us not just to want the good but actually to do good and not evil. Kant also talked about beneficence but left it up to the individual to choose when to apply it. According to Frankena the principle of beneficence has four "oughts": not to inflict harm or evil, to prevent harm, to remove evil, and to do or promote good.[13]

The principle of justice, distributive justice, is the equal or comparative treatment of individuals. Distributive justice seeks to distribute benefits and burdens equally throughout society. Criteria suggested as a basis to the exercise of distributive justice are: dealing with people according to their merits, treating people as equals in distributing good and evil equally among everyone, and treating people according to their needs.[14] One now has the problem of deciding which criterion to use.

These two principles of justice and beneficence may come into conflict at the individual action level and at the public policy level. Frankena seems to suggest that as we approximate solutions to ethical dilemmas in a cooperative effort these two principles will not be inconsistent. An example of trying to apply these principles at the public policy level might be the work of the interdisciplinary National Commission for the Protection of Human Subjects established by the National Research Act of 1974.

Ideal Observer Theory

Firth proposes a theory that he calls the "ideal observer" theory. This is a theory of cognitive processes. The qualities of consistency, disinterestedness, dispassionateness, omniprecipience, omniscience, and normality characterize the "ideal observer" or moral judge, which could be an individual or a machine, e.g., a computer. Omniscience means obtaining all the information one can about the situation in question. No limits are put on what the "ideal observer" should know. No information can be censored. Omniprecipience, a word coined by Firth, is the ability to see implications and consequences of projected actions as if one is experiencing them. One uses all one's powers of imagination to do this with the awareness that one can never totally enter into another person's experience. Some call this empathy.[15]

Dispassionateness and disinterestedness refer to impartiality. One is impartial in the sense that one has no particular interests or egocentric relationships in the given dilemma. The "ideal observer" only has general interests such as the welfare of all and does not experience emotions of jealousy, self-love, or any similar emotions directed to particular individuals. To experience such emotions is to be disqualified as a moral judge. Impartiality also assumes equal treatment for everyone.[16]

The notion of consistency refers to ethical decisions made in two different situations. These decisions must be consistent with each other in the sense that any "ideal observer" would react in the same manner to a given act. Firth acknowledges that these decisions might vary with the culture. Consistency follows from the other qualities discussed in combination with recognized psychologic laws of behavior. In other respects, the "ideal observer" falls within the range of "normality."[17] He or she observes the physical and mental conditions favorable for making valid decisions, i.e., is not sick, hungry, cold, tired, or suffering from jet lag.

This theory provides us with characteristics of ethical reasoning and reflective thinking, but, again, does not make it easier to solve specific ethical dilemmas. However, it does provide us with some criteria for examining ethical dilemmas and alternatives for action from the point of view of an "ideal observer." It also provides some assistance to health professionals in deciding when they should *not* be the judge in a given situation and should seek the help of others, perhaps a committee. One might ask, Where will development of this moral conscientiousness occur? In what social institutions?

Justice as Fairness

Rawls discusses justice as fairness and as the foundation of social structure. Justice, broadly speaking, has to do with the distribution of good and evil, harms and benefits in society. His theory offers us another perspective from which to view ethical decision making and the basis for moral decisions. It is a rethinking of the social contract theory of obligation in the Kantian tradition. The heart of the theory is the notion of the "original position" in which people come together to negotiate the principles of justice by which all are bound to live. According to Rawls, the principles of justice have to do with distribution of what he calls primary goods: income, wealth, liberty, opportunity, and the bases of self-respect. The negotiators are rational, intelligent people who wish to pursue their own goals in a just society.[18]

Rawls places the negotiators under the constraints of a "veil of ignorance." They have general knowledge and facts about such areas as physics and economics. They do not know any particular facts about themselves or others, e.g., personal characteristics, sex, social class. The purpose of the "veil of ignorance" is to remove from the negotiations any possibility of individuals seeking their own interests at the expense of others. This is the situation referred to as the "original position." The negotiators must favor only those principles that advance everyone's best interests. One might turn out to be one of the least advantaged individuals in a given community.[19] In the end, the negotiators must arrive at what Rawls calls "justice as fairness" because they do negotiate behind the "veil of ignorance."

The concept of "justice as fairness" is articulated in two basic principles of justice: (1) Each person is to have an equal right to the most extensive system of liberty for all, and (2) social and economic inequalities are to be arranged so that they are to the greatest benefit of the least advantaged and attached to offices and positions open to everyone under conditions of equality of opportunity.[20] The first principle, maximizing liberty for all, has absolute priority over the second if and when the two principles conflict.

Rawls also discusses five criteria for looking at the rightness of any ethical principles: (1) universality, i.e., same principles must hold for everyone, (2) generality, i.e., they must not refer to specific people or situations such as my mother or your marriage, (3) publicity, i.e., they must be known and recognized by all involved, (4) ordering, i.e., they must somehow order conflicting claims without resort to force, (5) finality, i.e., they may override the demands of law and custom.[21] Ethical egoism is ruled out as a standard for making ethical judgments by these criteria. A nurse could use these criteria to look at his or her own principles and values, those proposed by another health professional, or those assumed in a policy for a health care delivery model.

In considering justice as fairness inequalities are allowed only to improve the condition of the least advantaged, e.g., the retarded, children, the elderly. The least advantaged are in the normative position in society. Basic rights and obligations proceed from the notion of fairness for these disadvantaged groups. Vaux says this is invoking the "golden rule" in such a way that one is truly committed to the well-being of the other.[22] Justice as fairness to the least advantaged becomes the categorical imperative in the Kantian tradition.

Rawls makes no claim that his theory can be applied in contemporary society. Yet some critics raise objections to his work concerning his notions of primary good and the original position as if it did apply. However, he has provided us with a new way to look at moral problems in society generally and specifically in health care. How might the health care system look if the needs of the least advantaged were considered first in a public policy decision on allocation of health manpower resources?

The contemporary ethical positions discussed can be accepted or rejected on a variety of grounds as plausible ways of looking at ethical dilemmas in health care. See Table 1 for a summary of ethical positions discussed.

One finds any of these positions or a combination of them represented in health care settings whether or not an individual or group examines the assumptions or value positions underlying particular actions. There are difficulties in appealing to any one position for "the answer" to complex moral problems arising on the continuum from individual nurse–patient–colleague relationships to policy making for a neighborhood health center or the community at large.

Vaux provides us with a model for ethical reasoning and decision making developed from various moral positions. This model based on three "sources of ethical insight," human perceptions of past, present, and future, suggests questions that should be considered in any situation requiring an ethical decision. The first source is "retrospective insight" providing biologic, historical, religious, and philosophical views of the meaning and value of human life. The second source is "introspective insight" providing a look at life situations as they exist in the present. Values develop from these situations related to particular persons and acts occurring in particular times and circumstances.

Table 1. SUMMARY OF SELECTED ETHICAL THEORIES

Theory	Right-Making Characteristics
1. Egoism	One should do what will promote his own greatest good.
2. Deontology or formalism	One should consider other features of an act or rule than just its consequences.
3. Utilitarianism	One should consider greatest possible balance of happiness over unhappiness for the greatest number—implies that good and evil can be measured and balanced in some way.
4. Obligation: beneficence and justice (Frankena)	One should consider rules and actions from the basis of principles of beneficence and justice as equality.
5. Ideal observer (Firth)	One should consider actions and rules from a disinterested, dispassionate, omniprecipient, omniscient, consistent point of view.
6. Justice as fairness (Rawls)	One should consider rules and actions from point of view of least advantaged in society.

Third is "prospective insight," which considers the consequences of particular actions on man's possibilities and his future. Possible results on persons involved, side effects, and responses to a given action should be evaluated.[23]

These three sources of ethical insight represent factors that intersect in any ethical dilemma. The following questions emerge from these sources. First, what can be learned from the past that is relevant to this situation (e.g., Nuremberg)? Second, what do conscience and common sense demand in the present living situation? What makes sense for everyone concerned in this dilemma (e.g., tension involved in decision to have an abortion)? Third, what are the probable consequences of this or that action for the future (e.g., recombinant DNA research)?[24] It is the obligation of health professionals and others involved to consider all of these questions as a data base from which to make rational, thoughtful decisions in the face of complex ethical dilemmas. Echoes of all the ethical positions and theories discussed can be heard in these questions. Nurses, both as individuals and in collaboration with others, need to consider these questions in order to gather their own data bases to resolve the question of what is the morally right thing to do in a given situation.

Nurses might also take a look at recurrent ethical dilemmas and begin to wonder if they are all inevitable. Perhaps some dilemmas could be prevented from occurring at the primary level of prevention through listening, careful assessment, and education in colleague, patient, and family relationships. Ethical issues such as truth telling and experimentation with human subjects may well lend themselves to a preventive approach.

REFERENCES

1. Callahan D: Normative ethics and public morality in the life sciences. The Humanist, September/October 1972, p 5
2. Frankena WK: Ethics, 2nd ed. Englewood Cliffs, NJ, Prentice-Hall, 1973, p 19
3. Ibid, p 25
4. Ibid, p 24
5. Ross D: What makes right acts right? In Sellars W, Hospers J (eds): Readings in Ethical Theory. Englewood Cliffs, NJ. Prentice-Hall, 1970, pp 484–85
6. Frankena: op cit, p 29
7. Ibid, p 30
8. Kant I: The Metaphysical Elements of Justice, The Metaphysics of Morals, Part I. Indianapolis, Bobbs-Merrill, 1965, p 22
9. MacIntyre A: A Short History of Ethics. New York, Macmillan, 1966, p 195
10. Ibid, p 198
11. Frankena: op cit, pp 39–41
12. Ibid, pp 42–43
13. Ibid, p 47
14. Ibid, p 49
15. Firth R: Ethical absolutism and the ideal observer. In Sellars W, Hospers J: op cit, pp 212–14
16. Ibid, pp 214–18
17. Ibid, pp 218–21
18. Rawls J: A Theory of Justice. Cambridge, Massachusetts, Harvard University, 1971, pp 17–22, 62, 136–47
19. Ibid, pp 136–42
20. Ibid, p 302
21. Ibid, pp 131–35
22. Vaux K: Biomedical Ethics: Morality for the New Medicine. New York, Harper & Row, 1974, p 42
23. Ibid, pp 38–39
24. Ibid, pp 38–43

3

PROFESSIONAL ETHICS AND INSTITUTIONAL CONSTRAINTS IN NURSING PRACTICE

INTRODUCTION

As far as we can glean from history, the establishment of the first hospital occurred in India before the birth of Christ. Not until the Middle Ages did such institutions develop in Europe. As long as the sick remained at home, their care naturally fell to their families. But with the shift from the home to the hospital, the services of some attendants, in addition to the physicians, to care for the sick became a necessity. Early on in this development, two problems regarding these attendants received consideration: (1) how to secure nurses who would provide devoted service and (2) how to train them to give this service in an efficient manner. The first concern reflects a matter of ethical or religious ideals while the latter reflects a scientific objective. These considerations, in turn, involved many questions concerning the relationship of nurses to patients, on the one hand, and the relationship of nurses to physicians, on the other hand. Both considerations for ethical ideals and scientific objectives, along with the attendant questions regarding the nursing role and how it interacts with the other roles, such as patient and physician, remain with us today.

In the early development of these hospital attendants, who would evolve into the nursing professionals we know today, it is unclear whether they were thought of as glorified servants or whether they were viewed as professional personnel. In all probability a mixture of both attitudes coexisted and created a confusion regarding role and function that persisted through many later periods. Women, who constitute over 95 percent of nurses today in the United States, did not enter nursing at this earlier period. The fact that the first nurses were men has been explained by the generally inferior status of women at that time in those places where hospitals developed.[1] The status of women still remains a factor today, one that continues to affect nursing in some crucial ways.

Our knowledge of nursing generally goes back to the growth and spread of Christian influence in Europe. At that time the Church held nursing in high regard and made this known by bestowing sainthood on the nursing leaders. Later, in the sixteenth century, secular trends in nursing began to evolve. The paucity of scientific medicine made the situation such that nurses required no training beyond what could be gained by experience as they worked in the hospital. Nursing practice was, more often than not, a matter of difficult and unpleasant routines. In the past religious devotion had ennobled this toil and made it worthwhile, but now the religious basis for nursing practice was lacking. For more than three centuries after the Reformation, secular nursing carried with it no promise of a respectable career and the so-called better types of women tended to avoid it. For many years nursing was best described as a poorly paid, confining discipline of unpleasant routines, and the typical nurse was depicted as Sairey Gamp, the unpleasant, uneducated, uncouth character in Dickens' *Martin Chuzzlewit,* published in 1844.

The history of nursing in England and the United States since the mid-nineteenth century has evolved from the reforms that Florence Nightingale instituted in nursing education and practice. She maintained that a nursing school should teach the mind as well as form the character. The latter resulted in indoctrination and practice in the middle-class values of the period. Many remnants of the Victorian era and some strands from earlier times remain with us today and reflect the checkered history of nursing, which has included the image of both the saint and of the immoral prostitute. One historical study examining early American nursing points to another factor that has greatly affected the profession. This factor, the systematic oppression of the nursing profession, has affected the quality and delivery of health care.[2]

This chapter focuses on the nature of professional ethics in nursing and some of the institutional and social constraints which can act to inhibit the ethical practice of nursing. The discussion will be generally limited to those nurses who practice in hospitals for two reasons. First, we have more data on this group and, second, over 75 percent of all employed nurses work in hospitals.

NURSING ETHICS—A BRIEF BACKGROUND

Many books on nursing ethics in the past have in large part restricted their content to professional etiquette. In 1900 Robb wrote of a breach of etiquette, but her comments reflect the sociology of the situation, including differences in role, function, and status. She remarked that occasionally we find a nurse who, through ignorance or from an increase of her self-conceit and an exaggerated idea of her importance, may overstep the boundary in her relation with the doctor and commit some breach of etiquette. The point being driven home here is that not only will the individual nurse be made to suffer most acutely but also her school and the profession at large come in for a share of criticism and blame.[3]

Aikens in 1937 devoted two chapters to what she called old-fashioned virtues and included in this category such items as truth in nursing reports, discreetness of speech, obedience, being teachable, respect for authority, discipline, and loyalty.[4]

Perhaps one of the most interesting books on nursing ethics published as a fourth edition in 1943 has a chapter entitled "Master and Servant: Physicians and Nurse." The author says that if the hospital employs the nurse then she is a servant of the hospital and as such the hospital becomes responsible for her acts. With this status any disobedience to the physician's orders is not only a matter of professional etiquette but a violation of the employee contract. In those situations where the nurse knows that the physician is mishandling the patient's treatment she must either continue to carry out his orders or give up the case. This latter choice seems to reflect the fact that many nurses at the time this book was written worked as private duty nurses. The author continues by pointing out that the nurse has no duty to enlighten the public on the relative merits of physicians and the value of their treatment. In short, the nurse ought to remember that she has "a duty of charity as a faithful servant to a master to protect the good name and reputation of the physician under whom she works."[5]

Some years later another author quoted a remark made by a physician to a nursing school graduating class in which he said that to be a successful nurse, one must also be a successful liar. This quote led the book's author into a discussion of loyalty as the nurse's first duty. By virtue of her profession as well as of her implied contract, the nurse owes the physician not only efficient care of patients but also such evidence of loyalty as will strengthen the patient's confidence in him.[6]

All of the above references on nursing ethics were written in this century and many practicing nurses today read these books or ones similar to them when they were students. Among other things, such input reflects the nature of the socialization process into nursing, the role of women and nurses, and the hierarchical organization in the health care system. Many of these early ethics books delved into the private life and morality of nurses, reflecting the status of nursing students in an apprenticeship system and the stereotype of the intellectually and morally weak woman. Such concerns focused on the individual's morality and the nurse's duties, obligations, and loyalties refer to a situation in which nurses, on the one hand, were expected to exhibit a dedication of almost a religious nature while, on the other hand, they were open to suspicion regarding their morality.[7]

THE NURSING CODE OF ETHICS

The flavor of recent publications reflects some changes in the situation, but also some threads of continuity from these earlier concerns. The American Nurses' Association code of ethics outlined in Chapter 1 makes it clear that the nurse's primary commitment is to the patient's care and safety. In order to fulfill this commitment, the ANA maintains that the nurse must be alert to any instance of incompetent, unethical, or illegal practices by any member of the health team and must be willing to take appropriate actions if necessary. As to her own nursing practice with regard to fulfilling this commitment, the nurse has the personal responsibility of maintaining competence in practice throughout a professional career. In addition, if a nurse does not believe herself to be competent or adequately prepared to carry out a specific function, then she has the right and responsibility to refuse in order to protect both herself and the client.

Any such professional code must, by its very nature, address the general and the ideal, but in doing that it brings to the attention of practitioners the areas of ethical responsibilities, possible areas of ethical conflict, and potential mechanisms for coping with such conflict. In dealing with the general and the ideal rather than the specific and the concrete, a code can only allude to the formal and informal social systems in which practitioners function. For example, one recent sociologic study examined the norms involved in the phenomenon of how doctors in hospitals deal with evidence of error and incompetence among their colleagues. Essentially certain social mechanisms in the hospital work to cover up such mistakes.[8]

Taking into account historical factors and present realities, four central questions underlie the discussion in the remainder of this chapter. First, can nurses, employed in the bureaucratic system of the hospital, be ethical as outlined in the ANA code? Second, if they practice according to these ethical principles, do they run any risks and if so, what are they? Third, do nurses have the right as well as the obligation to provide adequate, if not excellent, nursing care and are they willing and able to exercise this right? Finally, what can the nurse expect from nursing in the way of support if she takes an ethical stance that disrupts some aspect of the hospital norms? These questions will serve to weave together the ideas in the next section on possible constraints which can function at times to inhibit ethical behavior on the part of nurses.

ORGANIZATIONAL AND SOCIAL CONSTRAINTS

One of the most interesting dimensions of hospital nursing arises in the potential for conflicting moral claims on the nurse. Until around the time of the Second World War, many, if not most, nurses in hospitals worked as private duty nurses and received a fee-for-service from the patient. A number of economic and sociologic factors converged in the 1930s and 1940s and this shift away from fee-for-service to hospital employee status occurred. Whereas previously the nurse's obligation had been to the one patient and the patient's physician, with this change in occupational status, the sociology and the ethics of the situation became more complex. As a hospital employee she must now balance loyalties to the institution, to the attending physician and the house staff, and to the patients themselves while attempting to practice nursing using the ethical code of the profession as a guideline.

Research in the past indicated that nurses believed that their first loyalty belonged to the hospital where they worked. By and large the potential ethical issues emerging from this situation went without discussion. In the last twenty years numerous members of the health professions and social scientists have described the roles, role expectations, functions, and status positions of those working in hospitals as well as the social network within which these workers function. Much has been said about the interpersonal and communication problems that arise, but a great deal less has been said about ethical dilemmas except indirectly, as they spin off from organizational, interpersonal, and communication problems.

One such study which examined baccalaureate students' images of nursing reported that these students, influenced by faculty, come to gravitate perceptibly toward individualistic-innovative views of nursing and away from bureaucratic orientations.[9] In a collection of essays a sociologist describes the physician as one who has a number of different positions that simultaneously provide him with multiple statuses and freedoms from organization control; however, he does have a quasi-contractual relationship with the hospital. The sheer power stemming from the free movement accorded to the physician within an otherwise formal bureaucracy sharply contrasts with the role of the nurse, which is profoundly affected by her obligation to represent continuity of time and place. Although the patient-care unit becomes her turf, the nurse and the doctor both know that in any direct conflict between them they will be subject to unequal privilege within the system. The implicit threat of the doctor's use of the free-flowing communication prerogative puts the nurse in a position of having to use flattery, tact, or even subterfuge in her role of co-ordinator between the entrepreneur and the bureaucratic system.[10] In another essay, Esther Lucille Brown discusses the system as a deterrent to professional nursing. She notes a number of factors involved, including the downward communication of frequent orders, rules, and prescribed procedures issued by persons in authority; the inadequate channels for upward communication of plans, suggestions, and complaints originating on the lower hierarchical levels of nursing; the problem of limited lateral communication and psychologic isolation all tend to decrease initiative and motivation and encourage dependency, feelings of inferiority, and dissatisfaction.[11] More recently, the experiences of seven new nurses attempting to innovate inpatient care illustrated some of these problems. They found the nursing administration authoritarian and stifling to the extent that they seemed to hamper improvement in patient care rather than encourage it. These young women asked, When will nursing administrators let nurses practice as legally indicated in their state's Nurse Practice Act?[12]

In another long essay based on field research, the point is made that nurses help doctors in scientific tasks and also help overcome inadequacies in the scientific method of practicing medicine. Essentially, the nurse does this by helping to prevent knowledge concerning ambiguities, uncertainties, and errors from reaching the patient and his family. The nurse is expected to react with moral passivity to her knowledge of hospital events. If she were a full-fledged professional peer of the physician she would, conceivably, take a more active moral stand whereas now she serves more as a sponge and a buffer in the system.[13]

According to Emile Durkheim professionals are part of a moral community. They have social links not only to their clients and colleagues in their own profession, but also to other groups with whose activities their skills must dovetail. Furthermore, the legitimacy of their professional contribution must be acknowledged by these other groups.[14] By comparison to the professions, the semiprofessional organizations are more bureaucratic and subject to numerous rules governing not just the central work tasks but extraneous details of conduct on the job. Semiprofessionals do not have a strong reference group orientation to colleagues and do not tend to see the generalized colleague group as a source of norms. Therefore they become more willing to accept an administrative superior as such a source.[15] One reason for this pattern in the semiprofessions is the prevalence of women, who seem to be more amenable to administrative control than men, less conscious of organizational status, and more submissive in this context than men.[16] These constraints do not tend to make for job satisfaction and can compound the already existing ethical dilemmas. A recent survey illustrates this point. Out of 10,000 nurses throughout the country who responded to this survey, 3800 said that they would not want to be a patient in the hospitals where they worked.[17] Not only did these findings raise serious questions about the quality of hospital care, but also shocked some leaders of the nation's hospital industry. Specifically, the survey reported that 18 percent of the respondents said that they knew of deaths caused accidentally by nurses, and 42 percent said that they knew of deaths caused by doctors. Four percent of these nurses reported that they themselves had made mistakes that they believed had led to a patient's death. These findings raise a host of questions regarding the ethical issues in these situations. Such questions come to mind as, How were these situations dealt with ethically? Were formal and/or informal institutional mechanisms available to consider the ethical aspects of these problem situations?

One typical situation reported by a nurse told of a shortage of nursing personnel on the evening shift in the intensive care unit where the nurse had responsibility for six patients on ventilators in three separate rooms. This nurse spent about 15 minutes with one patient who was hemorrhaging and then returned to another room where the patient had accidentally disconnected himself from the machine, arrested, and died. This incident raised the question of human resources and staffing in an area where, by definition, critically ill patients require close attention. What obligation does the nurse have to voice her concern regarding the ethical and/or legal aspects of this situation? Where would she go with such a concern? Does the nursing service leadership have a moral obligation to try to prevent such an occurrence? One central question basic to all the others has to do with the nature and extent of the professional colleagueship that nurses have with one another and with the nursing service hierarchy. If one nurse raises questions that examine the ethical issues involved in a given situation who, if anyone, can she rely on for support in her attempt to practice according to the ANA Code of Ethics? What formal channels need she go through in order to have her concerns heard and seriously considered? At the core of these questions lies the larger question of whether hospital nurses have professional, colleagual relationships with one another and can such a social network function to provide an arena in which ethical dilemmas can be discussed. As part of this larger question the role of the nursing leadership must be examined. Given the bureaucratic structure of hospitals, what can the nursing service leadership do to implement the ANA Code of Ethics? How does this leadership view the obligations and rights of the staff nurse?

Another finding of this survey suggested that the doctor-nurse game, first described in print in 1967 by Stein, continues to be a factor in the daily routine and decision making.[18] One nurse put it this way: "The conflict itself is not so upsetting as the fact that the patient may have to wait hours or a day before the doctor eventually gets around to ordering what the nurse suggested should be done." This type of interaction has been documented in research. One in-depth study concluded that a lack of effective communication between doctors and nurses was a significant factor in explaining the poor patient care the researcher found. The nurses had power when it came to making decisions about their patients, but they never seemed to be giving advice to the doctor. The nurses pretended they never made diagnoses, although their diagnoses were crucial to the patients' lives. Nurses received no formal credit for their expertise from physicians or patients since theirs was the great informal power of the manipulative subordinate.[19]

Nurses perceive physicians as more deficient in communication and participation-encouraging behavior than in directive behaviors. The desired change in physician leadership patterns appears to require change not only in interprofessional behavior but also throughout the system of hospital organization.[20]

As a matter of fact, doctors do not enjoy a good reputation in their relationships with co-workers. They tend to regard others as working for them and not for the patient. Despite this delegation of tasks, doctors continue to feel a final medical responsibility, including ethical and legal aspects, for all that happens to their patients. Considerable evidence has been gathered to indicate that the doctor–nurse relation can be characterized by medical authoritarianism, on the one hand, and nursing's acceptance of dependence or even deference, on the other.[21] This has led one nursing leader to say that the most fundamental problem in nursing is its status as a woman's occupation in a male-dominated culture. Even the administrative positions in hospital nursing generally are available only with approval of the male-dominated systems in medicine and hospital administration. She goes on to say that nurses who strive to never make a mistake fail to realize that decisions that were never made can be just as wrong as those which were made incorrectly.[22] Wilma Scott Heide, a nurse and an ex-president of the National Organization for Women, agrees that the problems of nursing are symptoms of the oppression of women.[23] Bullough commented on this situation by pointing out that historically the subordination of women and the sex segregation of nursing and medicine helped to establish interactional patterns between the two professions that included subordination of nurses as well as informed doctor–nurse games. Reinforced by hospital training schools and the state laws that restricted the roles of nurses, these patterns led to stereotyped communication and interaction between nurses and physicians and this in turn has been a barrier to the full use of the knowledge and skills of nurses.[24] In nursing, those with ambitions for advancement tend to leave the bedside, since only by removing themselves from direct clinical involvement can they gain any feeling of autonomy.[25] Certain practice patterns such as primary care nursing seem to be changing this.

Brown views the situation in a similar but broader manner when she points out that the health services industry is unusual in that most of the skilled and unskilled workers are women, although the industry is largely controlled by men. Health service occupations are organized like craft unions, with rigid hierarchical separation and control by the top occupation. Conflicts occurring between men and women, between management and workers, often get played out as conflicts between occupations. Because this occupational and sexual segregation overlap, conflict usually revolves around the shape and structure of the occupation and can best be characterized as maneuvering for turf, or, put another way, for control of occupational territory.[26]

A number of factors come together to maintain the situation referred to above. In the past, nursing has drawn into its ranks young women who have had a traditional view of the female role. One study conducted at a top-ranking university school of nursing administered questionnaires to three entering classes and three graduating classes during the years 1962 through 1965. The picture that emerged was that of conventionally oriented young women, much more heavily invested in traditional feminine life goals than in career pursuits and reluctant to make more than incidental concessions toward professional involvement.[27] Such data point to the fact that the traditional female socialization remains a major factor in women's work role. It also helps to remind us that the work world is, for the most part, geared to men and not to women, who have different home responsibilities. It reminds us too that not only do we lack good child-care facilities, but also that men have been socialized to hold certain ideas about themselves and their wives regarding their respective roles both in the home and outside of it.

More recently at a 1975 research presentation, Hall reported on findings from a study in which she compared female nursing students with female medical students. Again, the study found the nursing students expressed a more traditional view of the female role and lacked a career commitment.[28] In short, up to the present nursing has mostly attracted women with a traditional view of their role and this has had serious consequences for nursing and has served the function of maintaining the status quo in the decision-making arrangements within hospitals. Some earlier studies also make this point regarding maintenance of the status quo.

In 1966 researchers designed and executed an experiment in nurse–physician relationships. They believed that the professional status and standards of nurses are challenged at times by the behavior of doctors. They selected the situation in which the doctor directs the nurse to carry out a procedure that, in some fashion, went against her professional standards. Specifically, they constructed an incident around an irregular order from a doctor to a nurse for her to administer a dose of medication. Essentially, the ingredients of the experimental conflict included (1) the request of the nurse to give an obviously excessive dose of medicine (since this was a "live" situation, they decided to use a placebo for reasons of safety); (2) the medication order was transmitted by telephone, a procedure in violation of hospital policy; (3) the medication was unauthorized, that is, a drug that had not been placed on the ward stock list and cleared for use; and (4) the order was given to the nurse by an unfamiliar voice. The researchers conducted this conflict situation on 10 wards of a private hospital and on 12 wards of a public hospital. One nurse per ward participated for a total sample of 22 nurses. Of this total, 21 nurses prepared the medication and were walking to the patient with it when they were stopped. In an interview following the conflict situation, a majority of the nurses referred to the displeasure of doctors on occasions when nursing resistance had been offered to instructions that had been considered improper. It has long been recognized that when friction exists between doctors and nurses it is the patients who chiefly suffer. However, this study underscores the danger to patients in unresolved difficulties of the nurse–doctor relationship even when little or no friction in the usual sense of the word is present. In a situation such as this experimental one, it would be assumed by some that two professional intelligences, the doctor's and the nurse's, were working to ensure that procedures would be undertaken in ways beneficial to the patient. This study raises some question about that assumption. The authors of this study concluded that a considerable amount of self-deception goes on in the average staff nurse. In nonstressful moments, when thinking about her performance, the average nurse tends to believe that considerations of her patients' welfare and of her own professional honor will outweigh considerations leading to an automatic obedience to the doctor's orders at times when these two sets of loyalties come into conflict.[29]

The official view of the nursing profession is that the nurse will habitually defend the well-being of her patient as she sees it and strive to maintain the standards of her profession. This study surely counts among its implications the idea that professional relationships between nurses and doctors may be such as to exert a limiting effect upon the nurses' resourcefulness and, in some cases, increase the hazard to which the patients undergoing treatment are exposed. The trust and efficiency that the nurses demonstrated in the above study are qualities that, in their place, can be of inestimable value to physicians and patients. Obviously, the nursing and medical professions need to find ways in which these and other traditional values can be reconciled with the nurse's fuller exercise of her intellectual and ethical potentialities.

In another study conducted in the late 1960s, young women entering the professional part of their university education in social work and nursing described themselves, the characteristics of a good nurse, and the characteristics of a good social worker. The nursing students described themselves as dependable, methodical, capable, and conscientious, with some tendency to be submissive and sustain subordinate roles. They believed that the nursing role called for someone described as industrious, methodical, and dependable, with an ability to submit and sustain subordinate roles while being cooperative, considerate, conventional, and adaptable. The social work students described themselves and the good social worker as independent, spontaneous, and assertive.[30]

Before completing this discussion on organizational and social constraints, special notice must be given to the concept of paternalism. In his essay *On Liberty,* Mill wrote "that the sole end for which mankind are warranted, individually or collectively, in interfering with the liberty of action of any of their number, is self-protection. . . . He cannot rightfully be compelled to do or forbear because it will be better for him to do so, because it will make him happier, because, in the opinion of others to do so would be wise, or even right." Essentially what Mill is saying is that we cannot advance the interests of the individual by compulsion, or if we attempt to do so, the evil involved outweighs the good done. Mill believed that the individual person could best serve as judge and appraiser of his own welfare, interests, needs, and so forth. Others, including fellow Utilitarians, have vigorously attacked this claim on the grounds that little proof exists to indicate that most adults are well acquainted with their own interests.[31]

Paternalism can be thought of as the use of coercion to achieve a good that is not recognized as such by those individuals for whom the good is intended. Because coercing a person for his own good denies him a status as an individual entity, Mill strongly objected to paternalism and in absolute terms. To be able to choose is a good that is independent of the wisdom of what is chosen or, as Mill put it, a person's mode of laying out his existence is the best, not because it is the best in itself, but because it is his own mode. Mill's position has some problems in it which remain beyond the scope of this discussion; however, for him paternalism became justified only to preserve a wider range of freedom for the individual in question.

The concept, paternalism, as used in the medical ethics literature, most often refers to the attitudes and behaviors of the physician toward the patient. However, Ashley, in her historical study mentioned earlier, documents that paternalism on the part of doctors has resulted in serious and systematic injustice against women in the health sciences that has been both morally indefensible and socially damaging. She develops her thesis by pointing out that medicine and nursing have not constituted a complementary pair of professional groups sharing common interests and goals. Although they developed in close proximity, this has not resulted in cooperative activity for the good of the patient. In large part this situation resulted from the paternalism in medicine; paternalism, in this case, laced with prestige and power. A recent event in Texas demonstrated the paternalism not only of medicine but of hospital administration. The Texas Nurse Practice Act allows anyone, with or without a license, to practice nursing if under the supervision of a physician. This situation would be corrected if the proposed rewritten act introduced into the legislature became law. In addition, the bill makes continuing education mandatory for relicensure. This has occurred or is under discussion in other states. The Texas Hospital Association opposes almost the entire bill and the Texas Medical Association opposes parts of the bill, both in part on economic grounds. This human drama includes the abrupt dismissal of a hospital nursing director who had been credited with developing one of Texas' model nursing-care–delivery systems. This action came after she had held inservice meetings with the nursing staff to discuss the proposed nurse practice act and had provided them with copies of the present and proposed bills. The hospital spokesman's statement, "Her termination was not based solely on her support of the proposed nurse practice act, as alleged," did not impress everyone. The State representative to the hospital's Advisory Council resigned due to the dismissal.[32] When even the director of nursing is so vulnerable in the hospital system, it becomes understandable why nurses do not always take positions, including those on ethical dilemmas, and also why nurses do not always receive colleague support from other nurses. This situation at times becomes compounded by the fact that many married nurses are not mobile and cannot move to another area in order to seek employment. Also, some nurses make their homes in small towns where alternative employment is limited. One would like to be ideal and think that such considerations do not come into play when confronting an ethical dilemma; however, that strikes a naive chord.

SUMMARY

Bergman says that nurses face ethical issues on two levels, the policy level and in daily practice. She stresses the importance of dealing openly with conflict situations and the need for mutual respect.[33]

This chapter has raised questions regarding the second level and has focused on the possible organizational and social constraints in hospitals that may act to impede the ethical practice of nursing. Several interrelated themes have been developed and include the role and social position of the physician and the nurse in the hospital's social system, the bureaucratic nature of that system, the role and power of the nursing leadership in the system, sexism, and paternalism. In addition, the traditional female sex role socialization, which may have been reinforced by nursing school values, favors passivity in many matters including those of an ethical nature. In the extreme it leads to the

Nazi mentality where one does a good job by simply following orders. All of these factors combine to maintain the status quo.

The crucial questions as to the nurse and ethical dilemmas are: Given these factors, can the nurse be ethical? Is one factor the task of becoming aware of the ethical, as well as the clinical, aspects of nursing situations? Does one need to think through one's own values and ethical stances? What in the system can assist the nurse to act on her values and ethical stances? Would a formal mechanism of staff discussion help? Could some structural mechanisms be developed to provide colleagueship within the nursing ranks and between the staff and the leadership levels? Do nurses have a right as well as an obligation to attempt to practice according to the ANA Code of Ethics? Do they want to invest that much? The remainder of this book assumes that nurses do want to be guided by moral considerations in their professional activities, and to that end the following chapters discuss some central ethical dilemmas and nursing practice.

REFERENCES

1. Shryock RH: The History of Nursing. Philadelphia, Saunders, 1959
2. Ashley JA: Hospitals, Paternalism, and the Role of the Nurse. New York, Teachers College Press, 1976
3. Robb IH: Nursing Ethics. Cleveland, Koeckert, 1900, p 250
4. Aikens CA: Studies in Ethics for Nurses, 4th ed. Philadelphia, Saunders, 1937, pp 74–92
5. Moore DTV: Principles of Ethics, 4th ed. Philadelphia, Lippincott, 1943, Chap 13
6. McAllister JB: Ethics with Special Application to the Medical and Nursing Professions, 2nd ed. Philadelphia, Saunders, 1955
7. Deloughery GL, Gebbie KM: Political Dynamics: Impact on Nurses and Nursing. St Louis, Mosby, 1975, Chap 9
8. Millman M: The Unkindest Cut: Life in the Backroom of Medicine. New York, Morrow, 1977
9. Davis F, Olesen VL: Baccalaureate students' images of nursing. Nurs Res, Winter 1964, pp 8–15
10. Mauksch HO: The organizational context of nursing practice. In Davis F: The Nursing Profession. New York, Wiley, 1966, pp 109–37
11. Brown EL: Nursing and patient care. In Davis F: Ibid pp 176–203
12. Genn N: Where can nurses practice as they're taught? Am J Nurs, December 1974, pp 2212–15
13. Katz FE: Nurses. In Etzioni A: The Semi-Professions and Their Organization. New York, Free Press, 1969
14. Simpson G (trans): The Division of Labor. New York, Free Press, 1960

15. Simpson RL, Simpson IH: Women and bureaucracy in the semi-professions. In Etzioni A: op cit, pp 196–265
16. Etzioni A: op cit
17. Hospital nurses in a poll report needless deaths. New York Times, Sunday January 9, 1977, p 21
18. Stein LI: The doctor–nurse game. Arch Gen Psychiatr 16:699–703, 1967
19. Duff RS, Hollingshead AB: Sickness and Society. New York, Harper & Row, 1968
20. Bates B, Chamberlin RW: Physician leadership as perceived by nurses. Nurs Res, November–December 1970, pp 534–39
21. Bates B: Doctor and nurse: changing roles and relations. New Engl J Med, July 16, 1970, pp 129–34
22. Cleland V: Sex discrimination: nursing's most pervasive problem. Am J Nurs, August 1971, pp 1542–47
23. Heide WS: Nursing and women's liberation: a parallel. Am J Nurs, May 1973, pp 824–27
24. Bullough B: Barriers to the nurse practitioners movement: problems of women in a women's field. Int J Health Serv 5:225–33, 1975
25. ——, Bullough VL: Sex discrimination in health care. Nurs Outlook, January 1975, pp 40–45
26. Brown CA: Women workers in the health service industry. Int J Health Serv, 5:173–84, 1975
27. Davis F, Olesen VL, Whittaker EW: Problems and issues in collegiate nursing education. In Davis F: The Nursing Profession. New York, Wiley, 1966, pp 138–75
28. Hall B: Comparative study of female nursing students and female medical students. Paper presented at the Western Interstate Council of Higher Education in Nursing Research Conference, Phoenix, Spring, 1975
29. Hofling CK et al: An experimental study in nurse–physician relationships. J Nerv Ment Dis 143:171–80, 1966
30. Davis AJ: Self-concept, occupational role expectations and occupational choice in nursing and social work. Nurs Res; January–February 1969, pp 55–59
31. Hart HLA: Law, Liberty and Morality. Stanford, Calif, Stanford University Press, 1963
32. News. Am J Nurs, April 1977, p 534
33. Bergman R: Ethics—concepts and practice. Int Nurs Rev, September–October 1973, pp 140–41, 152

4

RIGHTS OF PATIENTS IN THE HEALTH CARE SYSTEM

INTRODUCTION

Rights of individual persons emerge within the relationships of a human community. Our society has changed dramatically during the past two centuries from a society that emphasized the obligations of citizens to one that focuses primarily on rights of citizens and the protection of these rights. The list of rights claimed in today's world is almost endless: the rights to privacy, to life, to death, to a healthy environment, to health, rights of children, the mentally retarded, the fetus, and the pregnant woman. This swing from citizen obligations to rights may be traced to a fear of the growing power of the social and economic systems and our increasing dependence on faceless organizations.[1] Jellinek says that patient trust is eroded in large impersonal medical centers and gives numerous examples of this in patient–institution relationships and arrangements such as lack of continuity of care and frequent violations of confidentiality.[2]

Respect for individuals within a social context underlies the notion that individual persons have rights. But where do rights come from and what are they? One view of rights says that individuals derive rights from natural law, which has its source in the Greek tradition of justice. This is the law of the cosmos, necessary, inevitable, and eternal. The divinely ordered Platonic universe eventually merged with the Judaic concept of the world and natural rights created by God, the law giver. Natural law as a source of rights, rejected for the most part by the modern world, says that there are natural, universal, and inalienable rights of men as a part of nature.[3] The origin of rights in this tradition is not clear except to say that they have their origins in natural law, i.e., nature. The only way to know what these alleged natural rights are is through the use of human reason. This provides no way to settle disputes when one person's reason conflicts with that of another.

The modern world view, denying that there are natural rights per se, maintains that rights are derived from the state and ordered by law. Such documents as the United Nations Declaration of Human Rights claims that there are fundamental human rights, including health-related rights, that all people should enjoy. However, the simple assertion of rights does not mean they exist in the legal sense and are exercised in society.

It is difficult to get a handle on the meaning of rights from dictionary definitions. Rights are defined in *Webster's Third New International Dictionary* as privileges, as just claims, doing what is just or good, one's prerogative, and power or privilege to which one is justly entitled. One does get the impression that rights are somehow entwined with a given social system and its legal subsystem. However, we still do not have a clear notion of what we are talking about when we use the term *rights*.

Within a legal system a right has to do with the power and control of an individual to change something or to keep it the same, e.g., a relationship. Distinguishing rights from claims, because they are often confused, Curran suggests that a claim is a right against another person either in the sense of one's person or property. One example is an individual's rights not to be assaulted by a physician while receiving medical treatment.[4] The other end of a claim is duty or obligation. In the example given, the physician has the obligation not to assault the patient. A privilege is a benefit, advantage, or immunity given to you by someone else, e.g., joining an exclusive club. In claiming a right within the legal system, one must seek an answer to the question whether or not something is actually endangered.

The Constitution of the United States puts forth what people may broadly expect from the federal government, e.g., purposes and functions of government, relationships with state governments, and some notion of what individuals must relinquish in order to preserve the interests and safety of everyone. Constitutional amendments speak more distinctly to rights of protection of individuals or groups from governmental interference, providing citizens with a very broad sweep of rights. Constitutional amendments are appealed to in cases where rights of citizens are challenged, as in the case of civil rights, for example.

Macklin, a philosopher, maintains that some of the debates and uncertainties about rights would be resolved to some extent if we had a framework provided by an overall theory of justice. One example might be Rawls' theory of justice as fairness. Lacking a social consensus on an overall theory of justice, it is difficult to justify specific rights. However, claims to rights may still serve "as expressions of moral outrage or as demands for social and legislative reform."[5] This use of the term "rights" is demonstrated in legislation of patient rights in the states of New York and Minnesota and in California's Natural Death Act (1976).

In asserting certain rights in the area of applied ethics, e.g., medical ethics, one must recognize that this is only one way of placing issues within an ethical framework. One may also consider the deontologic approach, which stresses duties and obligations, or the utilitarian approach, which looks at consequences of actions in terms of utility and the greatest good for the greatest number. Sometimes framing an issue in terms of rights only confuses the issue further. This is the case when, for example, individual rights that are difficult to substantiate are claimed, such as the right to health. Another aspect of the confusion is that one can justifiably claim to possess a right even though that claim is currently unprotected by law or social custom. It may help to distinguish between realized and unrealized rights.[6] Szasz refers to unrealized rights as "claims" to something not recognized by society. Sometimes rights are translated into duties and obligations, e.g., a right to health care would imply that others should provide care to those who want it.[7]

Macklin warns that there are many moral and philosophical problems in the attempt to discover where rights come from and in whom they reside, even though they are so often appealed to in public debate and in making demands for action of a particular kind.[8] In relation to translating rights into obligations, she says that not all the obligations within the area of health care can be derived from the rights of some persons or groups of persons.[9] Macklin's point is well taken when one considers the ethical issues that arise when rights are in conflict in providing particular kinds of health care. Whose obligation is it when very expensive medical care is provided for a middle-class child and no care is provided to the child whose parents are poor? Can an obligation be derived simply from the poor child's need for care? Another example of obligations arising from sources other than rights of individuals or groups is in obligations of the nurse that arise from the knowledge base of the profession and from the fact that nursing provides a socially valuable service.

Hart, attempting to clarify the language of rights, distinguishes between special and general rights. Special rights are those that arise out of particular transactions or relations between persons in the transactions. In these transactions, rights and duties exist only between the participants, for example, the patient–physician relationship or child–parent relationship. General rights for

Hart are those that arise out of a principle of equity that all persons equally have the right to be free.[10] In situations where conflict of rights occurs, one person's freedom is necessarily limited by that of another. Everyone does not have free access to health care facilities, thus limiting the freedom of those who do not have access to certain levels of wellness or illness. Hart's position on rights still does not provide us with reasons or justification for making claims about rights.

For purposes of this chapter, following Macklin's thinking, the concept of rights will be used to indicate some legitimate expectations of persons in a given society at a given time. Claims about rights are not to be viewed as something to be discovered as true or false, but as language used to promote change and social and legislative reform. Rights do not assert anything about the moral order per se. Legally, rights are viewed, as mentioned earlier, as the power to change or not to change a relationship, not unlike the philosophical notion of rights in our society at the present time as language to promote change.

What of the claim that one has a right to health? Certainly, this is an unrealized right at the present time if it exists at all. We now turn to a discussion of rights and obligations in the arena of health and health care.

RIGHT TO HEALTH

If one claims the right to health, to whom does one present the claim? Physicians? Government? Health educators? Self? Is there a corresponding moral obligation on another's part to provide persons with health? One is hard put to find a definition of health to which one could make a claim as a right. The World Health Organization's concept that health is a "state of complete physical, mental, and social well-being" does not give much direction when considered in the light of rights, public policy, and the limitless economic burdens that its realization would entail for society. It becomes even more difficult to take the "right to health" seriously when one thinks of how many people are labeled as "sick" in our society. One thinks of a range of persons from the hospitalized individual to someone whose behavior we do not like. "Health" is a terribly slippery term even when one thinks of it in terms of absence of illness or ability to carry on daily activities. Presently, there is no legal right to health.[11]

Callahan suggests that the "right to health care" as a social obligation might be undertaken by a society in terms of equal access to available health care and facilities.[12] Even this concept has difficulties in terms of the competition of health with other welfare rights and in setting limits on kinds of health care available and to whom. Health per se is not always a top social priority.

For example, do children and the elderly have the same rights to health care? What about equal access to health care for those whose illnesses can be traced to particular life styles and poor health habits? The smoker and the obese come to mind. An additional complication to this issue is that no one can yet explain why individuals do have undesirable health habits.[13] Are the causes of undesirable habits, such as smoking, genetic, psychologic, and/or physiologic? No one yet knows.

Another possible solution to the dilemmas involved in health as a right is to talk about the right to health care or to medical care more narrowly. The former notion is embodied in the concept of legislation for national health insurance. The latter concept underlies Medicare and Medicaid. Sade, a physician, claims that medical care is not a right since man has a primary right, the right to his own life.[14] As a consequence of this right, physicians should not be coerced into government schemes that require their services. If a physician is forced to meet this governmental obligation, then he has lost personal liberty, the right to one's own life, and personal freedom to decide how one will practice medicine. This position seems to assume that physicians have no obligations to society even though society legitimizes their practice as a socially valuable service. It also assumes that only physicians will have freedom curtailed to some degree by making medical care a right or a matter of public interest. Again this position points up the conflict of rights between individuals and the welfare of all, that is, the right of the physician to practice medicine at his discretion versus the interests of society, rich and poor alike. This question is by no means settled. Various legal cases have occurred that raise the question about the physician's obligation to the public in treating certain individuals, for example, the duty to warn an individual who suffers seizures not to drive an automobile.[15]

If it is the obligation of government to provide health care, what of the obligations of individuals not only to obtain care but to consider the influence of their own personal habits on the maintenance of health? Several authors point out the problems of putting more money into medical care when more medical care is not the answer to many of the health problems in our present society, for example, alcoholism and automobile accidents.[16-18] These authors focus on the need for a balance between availability of more medical care and individual responsibility for health maintenance. Illich calls the dependence of individuals on the medical care system, its care and drugs, the "medicalization of life."

Sparer, taking a broad view of health, says that rights to health care and the fostering of health should include attention to such "preconditions" of health as general environmental conditions, e.g., clean air, clean water, housing and working conditions, income adequacy, and personal habits for promoting and maintaining health.[19] Again, these factors may be more important to the health of citizens than more medical manpower and health care facilities.

Fried proposes the more feasible economic possibility of making a "decent minimum" of health care available to all. However, he points out that this is relative to what is available over all and what the best might be.[20] There are individuals and families in our society who do not get needed health care, for example, the poor and the elderly. The promise of Medicaid to make quality care available for the poor has largely failed. The poor are still dependent primarily on outpatient clinics and emergency rooms of municipal and county hospitals.[21] The courts have affirmed a governmental obligation to furnish citizens with minimum "necessities of life" including health care.[22] Yet this does not mean equal treatment for all and is a far cry from Rawls' notion of justice, which says that the benefits and burdens of society should be distributed to the advantage and disadvantage of all in society. The least advantaged must always benefit in the distribution of benefits in society according to this theory.[23] One is reminded of Macklin's point that we have difficulty in determining what rights are and how they originate, because we have no overall theory of justice for a framework in which specific rights could be claimed and justified.

The problem still remains to determine what exactly constitutes a minimum standard of housing or health care. This is complicated by the development of "needs" that would have been considered luxuries a generation ago in our society. If one appeals to needs as a standard for making medical care available, whose needs serve as the criterion? Again, needs and demands represent two very different concepts in looking at claims to rights for care. Is the health care system obligated to meet demands as well as to provide care to meet needs? Who decides what needs are to be met in providing a "decent minimum" of health care?

Generally, under common law, there is no legal right to medical care for the public from private health care providers. However, the Manlove case in Delaware said that private hospitals do incur legal obligations to the community by offering care and having an emergency room. The hospital meets a public need and offers a public benefit.[24] This has been very difficult to enforce in reality. Even government involvement in the form of Hill-Burton funds and federal tax exemptions to hospitals does not necessarily assure every individual access to care in a particular hospital. Some states, such as New York, have adopted statutes that require general hospitals to provide care in an emergency situation. These statutes exist in only a minority of states.[25]

One way to have rights to medical care is through a private contract with a physician, hospital, or other provider for certain kinds of care. The patient offers money to the provider as his part of the contract. Unfortunately, even if one has health insurance, it does not cover all costs associated with medical care and insurance plans generally favor hospitalization rather than ambulatory care services. Serious questions related to this issue are being raised in public about the necessity of the number of certain surgical procedures, hysterectomies, for example. Meanwhile, it is difficult to obtain general out-patient care and even more difficult and expensive to have this covered by one's health insurance. These "legal rights" under contract have generally been more available to the middle class than to the poor. Another mechanism for claiming rights is through malpractice suits such as *Canterbury* v. *Spence,* in which the right to informed consent was upheld.[26]

In order to make the unrealized right to health care a broad public right, Sparer suggests the following steps:

1. development of a consumer movement in which consumers actually do dominate in health planning;
2. linking health planning with financial control over the flow of public monies in health care which the National Health Planning Act of 1974 fails to do in an effective way;
3. enactment of some form of universal health insurance coverage;
4. tax reform aimed at achieving progressive taxation;
5. new approaches to enforcement of "rights" that consumers would demand; and
6. reconsideration of the role of the public sector in provision of health care.[27]

Underlying these steps is the assumption that health care as a broad public right has general social consensus. Yet there still exists much confusion and questioning in this area.

Having considered various points of view on the right to health care and medical care from the basis of access to care and the duty of the provider, we now turn to the rights of patients after gaining entry into the health care system.

PATIENT RIGHTS

The movement for patients' rights came out of the Welfare Rights Organization and demands for rights for the disadvantaged in the late 1960s. The overall goals of what is called the Patients' Rights Movement have to do with quality of health care, the improvement of care, and making some impact on health care providers to change the system. More specifically, individuals are seeking more self-determination and control over their own bodies when hospitalized in a paternalistic/maternalistic system. In this area one sees clearly the tension between what professionals consider to be their rights to provide care in the way they feel it would be most beneficial to patients and the patient's right to self-determination; tension between professional judgment and patient demands. Confidentiality, informed consent,

and patient rights to receive and refuse particular kinds of treatment all reflect the conflict between duties and rights of providers and consumers. This
theme carries through all chapters of this book.

Patients are protected against assault and battery by the law of torts (injury or wrongful act); but when it comes to such areas as informed consent
and truth telling, the issues are not clear cut for any individual situation.[28]
For example, what does one actually tell the patient? How does one tell it?
What level of risk should be disclosed? The standard used is what the reasonable patient needs to know to make a decision about treatment. Who defines
reasonable patient? A physician? A committee? A family? A community?
The rights of patients to participate in decision making are particularly difficult to determine in the mental health area. Then how does one apply the
criterion of the "reasonable" patient?

A further problem to be considered in the area of patient rights is the imbalance of power in the patient–physician or patient–provider relationship.
This imbalance is obvious as well in the Statement of the American Hospital
Association of the Patient's Bill of Rights in the paternalism underlying some
of the statements. Traditionally the patient is in a dependent relationship
vis-à-vis the provider and the hospital with his role legitimized by the physician.[29] In most instances it is the physician who is the gate-keeper of the
health care system although this is changing slowly in some areas of primary
care. One does not have access without the physician's sanction. The patients'
rights movement seeks a new model for this relationship, one in which the
traditional physician–patient relationship becomes more of a partnership in
the attainment of health. This cooperative model has the potential for striking
the balance between patient duties and rights discussed earlier by Morison.
Informed consent is another mechanism for making the patient a more active
participant in dealing with both the certainty and uncertainty of medical
care and the lack of ready guarantees.

The American Hospital Association Patients' Bill of Rights (1972), reprinted
here, speaks to the institution's obligation to patients in promoting their
rights to certain kinds of care and consideration within an institutional setting.

AMERICAN HOSPITAL ASSOCIATION STATEMENT
ON A PATIENT'S BILL OF RIGHTS*

1. The patient has the right to considerate and respectful care.
2. The patient has the right to obtain from his physician complete
   current information concerning his diagnosis, treatment, and prognosis in terms the patient can be reasonably expected to under-

*Reprinted with permission of the American Hospital Association, 840 N. Lake Shore
Drive, Chicago, Ill. 60611

stand. When it is not medically advisable to give such information to the patient, the information should be made available to an appropriate person in his behalf. He has the right to know by name the physician responsible for coordinating his care.

3. The patient has the right to receive from his physician informed consent prior to the start of any procedure and/or treatment. Except in emergencies, such information for informed consent, should include but not necessarily be limited to the specific procedure and/or treatment, the medically significant risks involved, and the probable duration of incapacitation. Where medically significant alternatives for care or treatment exist, or when the patient requests information concerning medical alternatives, the patient has the right to such information. The patient also has the right to know the name of the person responsible for the procedures and/or treatment.

4. The patient has the right to refuse treatment to the extent permitted by law, and to be informed of the medical consequences of his action.

5. The patient has the right to every consideration of his privacy concerning his own medical care program. Case discussion, consultation, examination, and treatment are confidential and should be conducted discreetly. Those not directly involved in his care must have the permission of the patient to be present.

6. The patient has the right to expect that all communications and records pertaining to his care should be treated as confidential.

7. The patient has the right to expect that within its capacity a hospital must make reasonable response to the request of a patient for services. The hospital must provide evaluation, service and/or referral as indicated by the urgency of the case. When medically permissible a patient may be transferred to another facility only after he has received complete information and explanation concerning the needs for the alternatives to such a transfer. The institution to which the patient is to be transferred must first have accepted the patient for transfer.

8. The patient has the right to obtain information as to any relationship of his hospital to other health care and educational institutions insofar as his care is concerned. The patient has the right to obtain information as to the existence of any professional relationships among individuals, by name, who are treating him.

9. The patient has the right to be advised if the hospital proposes to engage in or perform human experimentation affecting his care or treatment. The patient has the right to refuse to participate in such research projects.

10. The patient has the right to expect reasonable continuity of care. He has the right to know in advance what appointment times and physicians are available and where. The patient has the right to expect that the hospital will provide a mechanism whereby he is informed by his physician or a delegate of the physician of the patient's continuing health care requirements following discharge.
11. The patient has the right to examine and receive an explanation of his bill regardless of source of payment.
12. The patient has the right to know what hospital rules and regulations apply to his conduct as a patient.

Many of these proclaimed rights are "legally" unenforceable and are already in some hospital charters. Gaylin makes the point that the AHA Patients' Bill of Rights reflects the paternalism practiced in the hospital setting and only gives back to patients the rights that hospitals have so long ignored.[30]

The introductory statements of the brochure stating rights of the patient at Beth Israel Hospital, Boston, Massachusetts speak of meeting "goals" and asks the patient's help in doing this. The statements are more personalized than those of the AHA statement and convey an educational message to patients. It also reflects to some extent the authoritarianism of the hospital setting where patients must be told to behave in ways they might take for granted elsewhere. The Beth Israel document also mentions the patient's obligations to the institution. The document is presented here for the reader's consideration and comparison with the AHA statement:

YOUR RIGHTS AS A PATIENT AT BETH
ISRAEL HOSPITAL BOSTON*

1. You have the right to receive the best care medically indicated for your problem regardless of your race, color, religion, national origin or the source of payment for your care.
2. You have the right to be treated respectfully by others, and to be addressed by your proper name and without undue familiarity. Your individuality will be respected, and differences in cultural and educational background taken into account. When you have a question, you may expect to be listened to and receive an appropriate and helpful response.

*Reprinted with permission of Beth Israel Hospital, Boston, Mass. 02215

3. You have the right to privacy. You may expect to talk with your doctor, nurse, other health worker or an administrative officer in private, and know that the information you supply will not be overheard nor given to others without your permission. In the Hospital, when you are in a semiprivate room, you can expect a sincere and reasonable attempt to keep all conversations private.

   When you are examined, you are entitled to privacy—to have the curtains drawn, to know what role any observer may have in your care, to have any observers unrelated to your care leave if you so request.

   If you are hospitalized, no outsiders may see you without your permission. Your hospital records are private as well, and no person or agency beyond those caring for you may be permitted to learn the information in your medical record without your specific authorization.

4. You have the right to seek and receive all the information necessary for you to understand your medical situation. You have the right to know the name of the doctor who is responsible for your care and the right to talk with that doctor and any others who give you care. You are entitled to know fully about the planned course of diagnosis and treatment (including explanation about each day's procedures and tests), and the prognosis or medical outlook for your future. You are entitled to seek and receive adequate instruction in self-care, prevention of disability and maintenance of health. You have the right to ask your doctor any questions that concern you about your health.

   You have the right to know who will perform an operation or a test and to receive a full explanation of the details in advance, in order for you to exercise your right to give informed consent or elect to refuse. If you agree to the diagnostic and therapeutic procedures recommended by your doctor, you may be asked to sign a consent form. If you refuse, you may expect to receive the best help that the Hospital can still offer under the circumstances.

   You have the right to request and receive consultation on your medical condition, if you desire it.

5. You have the right to know when students are to perform specific examinations or treatments that pertain to your care. Because this is a university hospital, a major teaching hospital of Harvard Medical School, you may come across doctors, nurses and other health workers in training. We believe that the presence of these young professionals and students adds to the quality of care. You have the right to a full explanation of any training program for students

before you agree to participate in it, and the right to refuse to participate, without prejudice to the attention we give you.

6. You have the right to full explanation of any research study in which you may be asked to participate. No research study is ever carried out on any patient without his or her informed consent. If you are asked to participate in a study, you have the right to refuse to participate; you will still receive the best care the Hospital can provide.

7. You have the right to leave the Hospital even if your doctors advise against it, unless you have certain infectious diseases which may influence the health of others, or if you are incapable of maintaining your own safety, as defined by law. If you decide to leave before the doctors advise, the Hospital will not be responsible for any harm that this may cause you, and you will be asked to sign a "Discharge Against Advice" form.

8. By Massachusetts law you have the right of access to your medical record. As a general rule, we do not recommend that you review your medical record in the midst of a Hospital stay because, while you are an inpatient, your medical record is incomplete; it serves more as a work-sheet for your physicians and nurses rather than as a clear-cut listing of the pertinent medical facts of your case. During your hospitalization we urge you to direct questions to your physicians and your primary nurse, but if you still wish to see your record you have the right to do so.

   Patients no longer in the Hospital and ambulatory patients wishing to review their medical records or to obtain copies may make arrangements by calling the Medical Record Department at 735-3701. There is a small charge per page for copies. For your protection, we require signed authorization and positive identification to release medical record information.

   If you have questions on the information you acquire from your medical record, they should be directed to your own physician.

9. You have the right to inquire about the possibility of financial aid to help you in the payment of Hospital bills and the right to receive information and assistance in securing such aid. Information given to the Hospital on your own finances will remain confindential.

10. We believe you are entitled to know whether any facilities recommended for your use are businesses in which those making such recommendation have a significant financial interest, such as nursing homes, pharmacies or laboratories. Beth Israel Hospital has no such financial interests in any off-site facility.

You Also Have Some Responsibilities

Please keep appointments, or telephone the Hospital when you cannot keep a scheduled appointment. Bring with you information about past illnesses, hospitalizations, medications and other matters relating to your health. Be open and honest with us about instructions you receive concerning your health; let us know immediately if you do not understand them or if you feel that the instructions are such that you cannot follow them.

You have the responsibility to be considerate of other patients, and to see that your visitors are considerate as well, particularly with regard to noise and to smoking, which can be annoying to nearby patients. Visitors are not permitted to smoke in patients' rooms, the solariums or other patient areas.

You also have a responsibility to be prompt about payment of Hospital bills, to provide information necessary for insurance processing of your bills, and to be prompt about asking questions you may have concerning your bills.

4th Edition, November 1976

Even if many of these rights are legally unenforceable at this time, they provide patients, families, and providers with knowledge of those specific rights that consumers might expect and demand. Annas reminds us that if rights are not exercised, they may be forgotten and violations of them become routine.[31] He warns that hospitals could become "human rights wastelands." Both consumers and providers must take vigorous action to promote and protect human rights in institutional settings.[32]

Annas' book, *The Rights of Hospital Patients,* an American Civil Liberties handbook, provides patients and their families with a starting point in learning more about rights that can and should be exercised not only by and on behalf of hospitalized children and adults but also individuals using the services of emergency rooms, outpatient clinics, and neighborhood health centers. This book also acquaints the consumer with hospital organization and rules and standards which hospitals must meet. The corresponding problem that consumers should recognize is always that of enforcement of the stated rules and standards.

Neighborhood health centers have also established patients' bills of rights and obligations, which demonstrates further the influence of the patients' rights movement.[33] Minnesota and New York have both passed laws mandating Patient Bills of Rights. While there are limitations in the legislation since, for example, these laws may be interpreted by some physicians as the only rights that need to be afforded to patients, they do serve one of the purposes which Macklin suggests in her article discussed earlier in the chapter. That is, "rights" language and the proclamation of those rights can be used to generate action by social institutions that might not otherwise occur.

While it is agreed in principle that patients do have rights, it is still not easy to define and protect them. Kelly states that even though the AHA Statement has received much publicity there is not much evidence that hospitals have carried through on the presumed intent at the patient level.[34] Implementation problems were discussed at the National Symposium on Patients' Rights in Health Care sponsored by the U.S. Health Resources Administration in Washington, D.C., in the spring of 1976.[35] Representatives from consumer, provider, and government organizations discussed the serious and frustrating problems of moving to implement patient rights. It was clear that both providers and patients know too little about what patients' legal rights are. For example, some physicians were surprised that there are states where patients do not have legal rights to see their medical records. Criticism and frustration about existing patients' bills of rights were voiced in such complaints as not including information about complaint mechanisms and not providing enforcement mechanisms for stated rights. Further, pessimism about enforcement of patients' rights is even more realistic when one hears that federal responsibility for implementation is fragmented among some nine agencies that form the interagency working committee on patients' rights at the federal level.[36] Some authors have said that implementation of patients' rights will require a major restructuring of the health care system and passage of legislation to make possible the enforcement of those rights.[37-40]

The reader may be wondering why all the discussion about legally enforceable rights. One wonders if there are any rights and obligations that are granted for "humanitarian" or moral reasons. All this talk about legal rights seems to reinforce Macklin's contention that the language of rights does not seem to help us much in dealing with ethical issues and dilemmas in health care. In looking at this discussion of rights from a moral viewpoint one might consider the framework provided by Kohlberg's stages of developing moral judgment in the individual. One might hypothesize that as a society we are more at the level of Kohlberg's Stage 5 than of Stage 6.[41] Stage 5 is the social-contract legalistic orientation, which generally has utilitarian features, that is, the greatest good for the greatest number. Aside from what has been agreed on in society constitutionally and democratically, right is a matter of personal values and opinion. The legal point of view is emphasized with the existing possibility for changing law through rational consideration of social utility. Outside the legal system, free agreement and contract provide the basis for obligation. The notion of a contract between provider and patient was discussed earlier as one way to rights to health care. This social-contract legalistic orientation is the "official" morality of American government and the Constitution, the basis for many rights obtained through the Courts.[42]

Kohlberg's Stage 6 is the universal ethical principle orientation, which is more similar to the deontologic position or formalism and appeals to ethical principles such as the golden rule and the categorical imperative of Kant. To know the right-making characteristics of decisions and actions one appeals to moral principles that meet the criteria of logical comprehensiveness, universality, and consistency. These are such principles as justice, of the reciprocity and equality of human rights, and of respect for individual persons.[43] Kohlberg's research subjects for development of these stages were individual males in cross-cultural studies. However, it may be that groups and communities reflect predominantly one stage or another as they are the individuals who form them. One might speculate what implementation of patients' rights would look like from a Stage 6 orientation of consumers and providers.

To leave the speculative and return to the concrete, we turn to consideration of the Patient Rights' Advocate as one approach to more effective implementation of patients' rights within the existing medical care structure. According to Annas, the advocate should be accountable to and representative of the *patient*. Many hospitals do employ patient representatives.[44] These are not patient advocates. They deal with nonnursing and nonmedical matters related to patient comfort and convenience during hospitalization. The patient advocate should have the following capabilities in order to fulfill the duties of an advocate: access to all the patient's hospital records, the ability to call in qualified consultants, active participation in hospital committees monitoring patient quality of care, ability to lodge complaints directly to the hospital director and the hospital's Executive Committee, ability to delay discharges, and ability to participate at the patient's request and direction in discussions of the patient's case.[45]

Several objections are raised to this role in the hospital setting. Objections are that it interferes with current medical practice, patients' rights are already protected through informed consent and peer review, and it is only a "band-aid" approach to a fundamentally defective health care delivery system.[46] Another problem or potential problem is that most patient advocates are employees of the hospital. Whose rights will take priority in a patient–hospital conflict in which the patient advocate is involved? Annas suggests that perhaps third-party payers or health departments could provide the advocate's salary to decrease problems in this area. He also admits that the patient advocate role is no panacea, but does provide a mechanism for not losing sight of patients' rights in a bureaucratic structure where paternalistic providers with their technologies often forget that patients have rights to self-determination.[47]

In summary, we have briefly considered some problems in the concept of a right, rights to health and health care, provider obligations, patients' rights, and to a limited extent, their obligations within the health care system, and one formal mechanism for helping patients assert their rights within the system. We now turn to a discussion of the ethical implications for nursing practice, focusing generally on the concept of patient rights.

ETHICAL IMPLICATIONS FOR NURSING PRACTICE

Nurses and physicians often maintain that they serve as patient "advocates." One would have to question exactly what they mean when they invoke the term because the majority of health and medical care providers are employed in hospitals in states where it is now necessary to legislate patients' bills of rights. One might ask what has been advocated for patients by the health professionals. For example, do they advocate following the doctor's orders? Many patients find hospitals, particularly large medical centers, impersonal and dehumanizing. The patient's individualism and autonomy are left at the hospital door. Dyck, in talking about the dying patient, says that patients may need advocates other than physicians and nurses. One reason for this is the traditional medical ethic that proposes that one should do all one can to maintain life for the individual patient.[48]

Nurses certainly need to take time to look at all the ways in which they encourage or discourage patient autonomy within the limits of safety both in the hospital setting and in other settings such as the home. What is appropriate nursing behavior with the comatose patient, with the conscious patient, and even more, with the ambulatory patient? As patients increasingly demand their rights, what is nursing's response? Is the individual just labelled as another "difficult" patient or family member? Kelly affirms that the nurse's direct responsibility is to explain nursing care and to provide health education, which of course is now spelled out in some state legislated definitions of nursing so that health education is a legal as well as moral nursing obligation to patients.[49] There are tremendous implications in this nursing obligation for helping the patient meet obligations for maintenance of his own health. This is a key area with ever shorter hospitalizations for many patients and individual health problems related to lifestyle.

Kelly's discussion of the patient's "right to know" is an excellent overview of the many areas in which nurses have ethical obligations to patients, as in research that involves human subjects, informed consent, and during the dying process. She points out that nurses, as well as patients, are taking risks if nurses choose to encourage and reinforce the exercise of patient rights to the possible extent of losing a job. As we have said before, if nurses choose to practice openly as responsible and accountable to the patient, there must be support systems for this kind of practice, that is, a collegial system. How long will ethical nursing practice be compromised by fear and by lack of formal colleague support? What difference does it make at the patient level of care? What are the implications at the policy-making level of institutions where nurses are employed if nurses are to teach patients about their conditions and the physician does not want this done? What would happen to the image of nursing and to the health care structure if nurses did become patient advocates? As Kelly points out, there are no legal answers to the dilemmas for nursing inherent in these questions. We might ask if nursing has to wait for the courts to tell us that ethical practice has legal sanction.

What if nurses formed a consensus and moved actively to Kohlberg's 6th Stage, the universal ethical principle orientation and, for example, actively practiced the principle of respect for the individual patient? What changes would have to be made in the bureaucratic structure and organization of work for this principle to be honored in patient care? At what cost? To whom?

The Pregnant Patient's Bill of Rights, reprinted here, offers nursing the opportunity to protect and exercise the rights of both mother and unborn child in the hospital and/or clinic where most babies experience the world for the first time.

THE PREGNANT PATIENT'S BILL OF RIGHTS*

1. *The Pregnant Patient has the right,* prior to the administration of any drug or procedure, to be informed by the health professional caring for her of any potential direct or indirect effects, risks or hazards to herself or her unborn or newborn infant which may result from the use of a drug or procedure prescribed for or administered to her during pregnancy, labor, birth, or lactation.

2. *The Pregnant Patient has the right,* prior to the proposed therapy, to be informed, not only of the benefits, risks, and hazards of the proposed therapy but also of known alternative therapy, such as available childbirth education classes which could help to prepare the Pregnant Patient physically and mentally to cope with the discomfort or stress of pregnancy and the experience of childbirth, thereby reducing or eliminating her need for drugs and obstetric

*Reprinted with permission of the Committee on Patient's Rights, Box 1900, New York, N.Y. 10001

intervention. She should be offered such information early in her pregnancy in order that she may make a reasoned decision.

3. *The Pregnant Patient has the right,* prior to the administration of any drug, to be informed by the health professional who is prescribing or administering the drug to her that any drug which she takes during pregnancy, labor and birth, no matter how or when the drug is taken or administered, may adversely affect her unborn baby, directly or indirectly, and that there is no drug or chemical which has been proven safe for the unborn child.

4. *The Pregnant Patient has the right,* if cesarean section is anticipated, to be informed prior to the administration of any drug, and preferably prior to her hospitalization, that minimizing her and, in turn, her baby's intake of nonessential preoperative medicine will benefit her baby.

5. *The Pregnant Patient has the right,* prior to the administration of a drug or procedure, to be informed if there is NO properly controlled follow-up research which has established the safety of the drug or procedure with regard to its direct and/or indirect effects on the physiologic, mental and neurologic development of the child exposed, via the mother, to the drug or procedure during pregnancy, labor, birth or lactation (this would apply to virtually all drugs and the vast majority of obstetric procedures).

6. *The Pregnant Patient has the right,* prior to the administration of any drug, to be informed of the brand name and generic name of the drug in order that she may advise the health professional of any past adverse reaction to the drug.

7. *The Pregnant Patient has the right* to determine for herself, without pressure from her attendant, whether she will accept the risks inherent in the proposed therapy or refuse a drug or procedure.

8. *The Pregnant Patient has the right* to know the name and qualifications of the individual administering a medication or procedure to her during labor or birth.

9. *The Pregnant Patient has the right* to be informed, prior to the administration of any procedure, whether that procedure is being administered to her for her or her baby's benefit (medically indicated) or as an elective procedure (for convenience or teaching purposes).

10. *The Pregnant Patient has the right* to be accompanied during the stress of labor and birth by someone she cares for, and to whom she looks for emotional comfort and encouragement.

11. *The Pregnant Patient has the right* after appropriate medical consultation to choose a position for labor and for birth which is least stressful to her baby and to herself.

12. *The Obstetric Patient has the right* to have her baby cared for at her bedside if her baby is normal, and to feed her baby according to her baby's needs rather than according to the hospital regimen.
13. *The Obstetric Patient has the right* to be informed in writing of the name of the person who actually delivered her baby and the professional qualifications of that person. This information should also be on the birth certificate.
14. *The Obstetric Patient has the right* to be informed if there is any known or indicated aspect of her or her baby's care or condition which may cause her or her baby later difficulty or problems.
15. *The Obstetric Patient has the right* to have her and her baby's hospital medical records complete, accurate, and legible and to have their records, including Nurses' Notes, retained by the hospital until the child reaches at least the age of majority, or, alternatively, to have the records offered to her before they are destroyed.
16. *The Obstetric Patient,* both during and after her hospital stay, *has the right* to have access to her complete hospital medical records, including Nurses' Notes, and to receive a copy upon payment of a reasonable fee and without incurring the expense of retaining an attorney.

Putting the Bill into practice is an opportunity to help an individual make knowledgeable choices in specific areas during a critical time of experiencing for the born and unborn. The pregnant woman is not a passive object to be acted upon as is so often the situation in existing health care structures. Nurses could again act on the principle of respect for the individual to encourage self-determination. The paternalistic/maternalistic attitudes and decisions based on "we'll do what's best for you and the baby" could evolve into a more cooperative decision making process to involve everyone concerned, including the father or others.

Fagin suggests an approach that may be a prior step to helping patients achieve their rights, that is, the achievement and exercise of nurses' rights.[50] Nursing tradition and history have focused on the responsibility and service of the nurse as a helping professional rather than on nurses' autonomy and rights. Fagin sees nurses' rights emerging out of human rights and women's rights. One's human rights ought to encompass creation of those situations to enhance "humanness," e.g., feelings, compassions, sympathies, and intelligence. Involved in women's rights are freedom of choice, equality, and respect for the individual. This does not mean asking for special privileges but the right to equal and full participation. Fagin says that nurses have clearly stated the right "not to do," but need to say more specifically what they will do within rights "to do," such as rights to the type of environment that allows for professional nursing practice and professional economic rewards, a work environment that minimizes physical and emotional stresses, the right to set standards of excellence in nursing practice, and to participate in all policy making that affects nurses and nursing care.[51] These rights must be exercised by nurses in order that nurses' rights not be lost permanently in the depersonalized bureaucracies where physicians provide the direct care that is perceived by the public as valuable but where nurses' care is often attributed only to the physician's orders.

One way to be responsible and accountable for nursing care is to demand rights for patient care as an essential service in hospitals, nursing homes, and other settings, both publicly and politically. Power and leverage for such action exist within the new definitions of nursing adopted in some states. It is up to nurses, individually and collectively, to support each other in making these definitions a reality in health care systems. Achievement of nurses' rights could also help patients to exercise their rights and to meet obligations for their own health maintenance.

To talk about nurses' and patients' rights without action to make them come alive is to give in to passivity and further dependence on others, a far cry from what nursing can and should be for nurses and patients. Nurses can and sometimes do exercise rights at the bedside, in homes, and at policy-making levels of institutions and communities. It should be the rule rather than the exception. Will we leave the issue of rights in the realm of an ethical dilemma or will we make decisions and take action to make paper rights become realized rights?

REFERENCES

1. Morison RS: Rights and responsibilities: redressing the uneasy balance. Hastings Cent Rep, April 1974, p 1
2. Jellinek M: Erosion of patient trust in large medical centers. Hastings Cent Rep, June 1976, pp 16–19
3. Macklin R: Moral concerns and appeals to rights and duties. Hastings Cent Rep, October 1976, pp 32, 34
4. Curran WJ: Lecture in Human Rights and Health. Harvard School of Public Health, October 5, 1976
5. Macklin: op cit, p 31
6. Gorovitz S, Jameton AL, Macklin R, et al (eds): Moral problems on a social scale: introduction. In Moral Problems in Medicine. Englewood Cliffs, NJ, Prentice-Hall, 1976, p 426
7. Ibid: pp 426–27
8. Macklin: op cit, p 32
9. Ibid: pp 35–36

10. Ibid: p 37
11. Sparer EV: The legal right to health care. Hastings Cent Rep, October 1976, p 39
12. Callahan D: Health and society: some ethical imperatives. Daedalus, Winter 1977, pp 30–31
13. Ibid: p 32
14. Sade RM: Medical care as a right: a refutation. New Engl J Med 285: 1288–92, 1971
15. Curran WJ: Legal extension of the physician's obligations to the public in the treating of individual patients. Am J Public Health 64:624, 1974
16. Morison: op cit, pp 1–4
17. Wildavsky A: Doing better and feeling worse: the political pathology of health policy. Daedalus, Winter 1977, p 105
18. Illich I: Medical Nemesis: The Expropriation of Health. Toronto, McClelland and Stewart, 1975
19. Sparer: op cit, p 39
20. Fried C: Equality and rights in medical care. Hastings Cent Rep, February 1976, p 32
21. Cantor NL: The law and poor people's access to health care. Law Contemp Problems 35:902, 1970
22. Ibid: p 907
23. Rawls J: A Theory of Justice. Cambridge, Harvard University Press, 1971
24. Wilmington General Hospital v Manlove, 54 Del. 15, 174 A.2d 135 (1961)
25. Sparer: op cit, pp 40–41
26. Canterbury v Spence, 464 F.2d 772 (1972)
27. Sparer: op cit, p 46
28. Haley J: Lecture in Human Rights in Health. Harvard School of Public Health, November 9, 1976
29. Bloom SW, Wilson RN: Patient–practitioner relationships. In Freeman HE, Levine S, Reeder LG (eds): Handbook of Medical Sociology, 2nd ed. Englewood Cliffs, NJ, Prentice-Hall, 1972, pp 315–32
30. Gaylin W: Editorial: the patients' bill of rights. Saturday Rev Sci, March 1973, p 22
31. Annas GJ: The Rights of Hospital Patients: The Basic ACLU Guide to a Hospital Patient's Rights. New York, Avon, 1975
32. Ibid: p 1
33. King Health Center: Your Rights as a Patient. New York, 1972
34. Kelly LY: The patient's right to know. Nurs Outlook, January 1976, p 27
35. Hollander R: Patients' rights still not established. Hastings Cent Rep, August 1976, pp 10–11
36. Ibid: p 11
37. Fried: op cit, pp 32–34
38. Cantor: op cit, pp 901–22
39. Mechanic D: Rationing health care: public policy and the medical marketplace. Hastings Cent Rep, February 1976, pp 34–37

40. Fuchs VR: Who Shall Live? New York, Basic Books, 1974, pp 148-51
41. Duska R, Whelan M: Moral Development: A Guide to Piaget and Kohlberg. New York, Paulist Press, 1975, p 47
42. Ibid: p 47
43. Ibid: p 47
44. Annas: op cit, p 209
45. Ibid: p 211
46. Annas GJ: The patient has rights, how can we protect them? Hastings Cent Rep, September 1973, p 9
47. Ibid: p 9
48. Dyck AJ: An alternative to the ethic of euthanasia. In Williams RH (ed): To Live and to Die: When, Why, and How. New York, Springer, 1974, p 109
49. Kelly: op cit, p 29
50. Fagin CM: Nurses' rights. Am J Nurs 75:82-85, 1975
51. Ibid: p 84

5

INFORMED CONSENT

INTRODUCTION

Any discussion of informed consent must be placed within a larger context regarding the moral justification of conducting research using human subjects. In much, if not most, biomedical research with human subjects, we usually assume that previous trials have been conducted on animals and that careful assessment of predictable risks in comparison with foreseeable benefits has occurred. Although the moral issues of using animals in research to better the human condition are worthy of our close attention, they remain outside the present discussion.[1]

In order to proceed with a discussion of why and whether we should conduct research using human subjects, some definitions will be helpful. Therapy refers to a class of activity to benefit an individual or member of a group. The person giving therapy has the intention of benefiting the recipient of the activity. Research, on the other hand, refers to scientific activity to contribute to the general knowledge in a field. Two subtypes of research can be identified. First, scientists conduct therapeutic research mainly for the benefit of the subject while also gaining knowledge. For example, the giving of a new drug to a cancer patient can be basically for therapeutic purposes while at the same time it can be a trial test for the drug. Second, scientists also engage in nontherapeutic research using human subjects to gain new knowledge. For example, an experiment deliberately introduces change into a given situation and then measures and compares the effect between the control group and the experimental group. The control group does not usually benefit in any therapeutic way from the research. The motivation of those in the control group to participate has not been for therapeutic benefit, but for remuneration or the advancement of science.

The moral justification for conducting research using human subjects can be approached from the ethics of good consequences. We all derive social benefits from research whether that benefit is immediately therapeutic to us personally or whether it affects us indirectly by affecting resources. Eventually, a procedure or a drug, after being tested on nonhumans, must be tested on some humans so that the knowledge gained can be used for the larger social good. In addition, serious harm would develop from not conducting research using human subjects since scientific advances would be greatly limited. When you think about it, many, if not most of the health care measures, both preventive and curative, that we now take for granted were once experimental and involved human subjects in their development. We can morally justify using human subjects by arguing from a utilitarian position of good consequences for the greater number of people.

Using the concept of justice, one can also develop a nonconsequential argument to support and morally justify nontherapeutic research. We, as a society, benefit from the risks that others have taken in previous experiments; therefore, is it just for us to reap these benefits without reciprocal action? The practical matter that in biomedical research a time arrives when only human subjects can provide the data needed must neither overshadow nor obscure the ethical dilemmas involved.

To morally justify the use of humans in experimentation does not eliminate all of the possible ethical dilemmas that can confront the researcher once such research gets under way. Such considerations as freedom of choice and coercion, rights of the individual and needs of society, the meaning of "the good," the problem of uncertainty in determining the risk–benefit ratio represent some of the more obvious dimensions of these ethical dilemmas.

Research experimentation using humans as subjects can be traced back to the beginning of recorded history. This early research, mainly conducted in an unsystematic fashion within the clinical practice context, lead to instances of patients receiving treatments whose value had not been established by controlled, well-designed clinical investigation. In the past, many instances of researchers and health care professionals, including nurses, submitting themselves as subjects in research projects have also been reported.

Few questions arose over the years with regard to these practices since it was assumed that the individuals being used for research purposes also benefited as the recipients of the knowledge gained in these experimentations. Although the late nineteenth century saw an acceleration in the systematic use of human subjects for research purposes, this activity did not lead to an exploration of the need for safeguards protecting these individuals. One notable exception can be found in Bernard's 1865 publication in which he demonstrated the need for research using human subjects and began to develop rules of ethical conduct to govern such an enterprise.[2]

Along with medicine, law gave little attention to the rights of human subjects in experimentation. In the mid-1930s the Michigan Supreme Court stated that experimentation, although important and necessary, must be undertaken with the knowledge and consent of the patient or someone responsible for him and such procedures must not vary too radically from accepted practice.[3] This broad generalization that the Court used to distinguish between rash experimentation with humans and systematic and ethical scientific research practice did not anticipate the grave concerns that arose in a few years from the Nuremberg disclosures. The atrocities perpetrated by German physicians in the name of clinical research during the Third Reich disturbed many scientists who then wanted ethical standards established on a world-wide basis to protect human subjects.

REGULATIONS AND HUMAN SUBJECTS

The Nazi experiments, so far outside the limits of what anyone would consider accepted medical and research practice, tended to be viewed by some as a terrible and tragic moment in history but separate from the general problem of protection for research subjects. Such a view obscured the fact that in principle, although perhaps not in the same magnitude, many similar moral issues had characterized research since the beginning of experimentation. The Military Tribunal, which tried the Nazi physicians, formulated a code of ethics that has profoundly shaped the ethos of the experimental aspects of post-Second World War biomedical research. The following excerpts from the code illustrate the general nature of this document. The code states that voluntary consent of the human subject is absolutely essential and the duty and responsibility for ascertaining the quality of the consent rests upon each individual who initiates, directs, or engages in the experiment. This personal duty and responsibility may not be delegated to another with impunity. The code also says that the experiment should be such as to yield fruitful results for the good of society, unprocurable by other methods or means of

study, and not trivial or unnecessary in nature. Furthermore, the degree of
risk to be taken should never exceed that determined by the humanitarian
importance of the problem to be solved by the experiment. During the course
of the experiment, the human subject should be at liberty to end his participation in the experiment if he reaches the physical or mental state where continuation seems to him to be impossible. Additionally, the scientist must be
prepared to terminate the experiment at any stage if he believes that a continuation of the experiment is likely to result in injury, disability, or death to
the experimental subject.[4]

The promulgation of other codes such as the World Medical Association
Helsinki Declaration of 1964, the American Medical Association Ethical
Guidelines for Clinical Investigation of 1966, the American Psychological
Association Code of 1972, and the American Nurses' Association Human
Rights Guideline for Nurses in Clinical and Other Research of 1975 focused
attention not only on the ethical dilemmas inherent in research activities but
also on the limitation of codes to deal with these dilemmas adequately. As
indicated in Chapter 1, codes, succinctly worded and devoid of commentary,
although useful as general guidelines, cannot cover every possible eventuality
and remain limited and subject to interpretation.[5] These codes of ethics made
it clear, however, that the professions recognized that self-regulation by investigators could not be relied on solely to safeguard the rights of human
subjects in experiments. This realization coupled with the growing awareness
of the limitations of codes led to the development of procedures to apply the
general moral principles contained in the codes. The procedures took the
form of formal evaluation of research projects by institutional review committees. In 1953, the National Institute of Health developed procedures to regulate research conducted at its clinical center.[6] In 1971, the Department of
Health, Education, and Welfare formulated its policy for the protection of
human subjects and at present these policies vest basic responsibility for the
protection of human subjects in institutional review committees.[7] Because of
the prominent role that the federal government has in funding biomedical
research, over 700 institutions have established committees to review research protocols. Such institutional committees in hospitals, medical centers,
and other such facilities around the country are in charge of initial reviews
of all research proposals and periodic re-review in order to ascertain that
each researcher has outlined the risks and benefits and that the subjects
have given their informed consent to participate in the study. Essentially,
the committee must determine that the rights and welfare of the subjects
are protected, that the risks to an individual are outweighed by the potential benefits to him and/or society, and that informed consent will be obtained by adequate and appropriate methods. These governmental review
standards, although worded in general terms, do detail the basic elements of

informed consent, thereby drawing attention to its importance. Such standards should assist the scientific community in preventing future abuses like those in several of the more dramatic cases from the past: the cancer immunology experimentation at the Jewish Chronic Disease Hospital in New York, the hepatitis experiment on mentally retarded children institutionalized at Willowbrook, and the Tuskegee syphilis study on Southern blacks.[8-10] These studies and others that received less media coverage serve to show the extent to which the scientific merits of research can be vastly overshadowed by the violation of basic ethical principles pertaining to human dignity and human life imposed on experimental subjects.

The institutional committees review research protocols at the local level while the National Commission for the Protection of Human Subjects of Biomedical and Behavioral Research, an interdisciplinary group established in 1974 to advise the Department of Health, Education and Welfare, investigates the ethical principles of, and develops guidelines for, human experimentation on a national level. An increasing number of publications have focused on the regulatory and review processes themselves and on the guidelines developed to be used.[11-18] This establishment of commissions and councils and the development of guidelines and regulations is viewed by some professionals as onerous and even dangerous because these activities may interfere with scientific advancement. Others, however, believe we require even more social control in these matters. They do not believe the present devices, including informed consent, protect human subjects enough from the ever-present potential for abuse.

INFORMED CONSENT

The scientist has the ethical obligation to provide disclosure of information that includes the proclamation of benefits, the warning of risks, and the discussion of quandaries in order to obtain a consent from the potential research subject. This consent must be based on the subject's understanding of the information to the greatest extent possible in order for him to be considered properly informed.

The concept of informed consent grew from the malpractice litigation of the 1950s such as *Canterbury* v. *Spense,* mentioned in Chapter 1, in which a young man became paralyzed following surgery and a fall. More specifically, it arose from legal cases where the patient's attorney had difficulty proving negligence on the physician's part when using the usual community standards of medical practice for comparison. The informed consent approach shifted the legal claim from a charge of negligence to one of battery because the patient would not have consented to the procedure had he known of the possible risk. Since the doctor had not completely informed the patient as to these possible risks and alternatives, the patient had not given his informed consent. Without effective consent, the physician had treated or operated upon the patient in an unlawful manner. This use of the informed consent theory helped the paitent's lawyer in these types of cases since other doctors did not have to testify as to community standards. Later, however, the courts determined that the requirement of informed consent would be measured by the community standards of medical practitioners.[19] The informed consent concept had by that time gained a firm hold both in medical practice procedures and in research experimentation.

Two studies published ten years apart provide some insights into the ethical dilemmas involved in informed consent.[20,21] In 1966, Beecher maintained that codes of ethics made the bland assumption that meaningful or informed consent was available for the asking, while in reality this very often was not the case. Although he concedes that consent in the fullest sense may not be obtainable, it remains a goal toward which every researcher must nevertheless strive. With this in mind, he reviewed 50 studies in which he found only two mentions of informed consent, 12 seemed unethical, and generally his data suggested wide-spread ethical issues, especially with regard to informed consent. Following the position of the British Medical Research Council, Beecher said that not only should all investigations be conducted in an ethical manner but in the publications it should also be made unmistakably clear that the proprieties have been observed. He believed that journals have a moral obligation not to publish unethical research, even those studies with very valuable data. Such a policy would discourage unethical experimentation. Beecher concluded by making the point that the ethical approach has two important components, informed consent and the presence of an intelligent, informed, conscientious, compassionate, and responsible investigator. The other study, by Barker, published in 1976, made note of the fact that in the past decade we have increasingly perceived a social problem in the abuse of human subjects in medical experimentation. Two major reasons have led to this general recognition that experimentation with humans is a subject for concern: the increased power, scope, and funding of biomedical research and changes in values that increased the emphasis on equality, participation, and the challenging of arbitrary authority. Barker and his colleagues conducted a national survey in which they found that whereas the majority of the investigators were what they called "strict" with regard to balancing risks against benefits a significant minority were "permissive" or more willing to accept an unsatisfactory risk–benefit ratio. In light of the fact that most institutions and the federal government now require that the human subject in an experiment or his guardian understand that some treatment is being withheld or something is being done for reasons other than immediate therapy and that they must be informed of any risks and must give consent voluntarily, Barker produced some interesting data. With regard to the issue of informed consent these data again revealed a minority with "permissive" views and practices, although that minority was smaller than it was for an unfavorable risk-benefit ratio. These data raise the question of how it happens that the treatment of human subjects is sometimes less than ethical, even in some of the most respected university hospitals. Barker answered this question by saying that these abuses can be traced to defects in the training of researchers, to defects in the screening and monitoring of research by review committees, and to a fundamental tension between investigation and therapy.

In another study, Gray interviewed 51 women who were, or just had been, subjects in another study to determine the effects of a new labor-inducing drug. His findings indicated that although all 51 women signed a consent form, 20 of them learned only from Gray's interview that they were research subjects. Among this group of 20, most of them did not understand that there might be hazards, that they would be subjected to special procedures or that they were not required to participate in the study. Indeed, four of the women made it clear that they would not have participated if they had understood and realized that they had a choice.[22]

McDermott labeled the kind of situation in which it clearly seems in the best interests of society that certain information be obtained as the hard core of the ethical problems in clinical investigations and informed consent. The fact remains that if the future good of society is to be served, there will be times when the investigators must make an arbitrary judgment with respect to an individual. He went on to say that if we followed the Helsinki Declaration and the Food and Drug Administration regulations to the letter we would have the curious situation in which the only stated public interest would be that of the individual since the future interests of society, at times in conflict with the interest of the individual, are ignored.[23] Many questions arise here such as, what does he mean by arbitrary judgment, which individual patients by age, sex, ethnic group, socioeconomic status will this involve, what are the interests of society, and by whose definition?

For most authorities on the matter, the core of the informed consent process is the balancing of risks to the human subject against possible benefits to him and/or society. However, Jonas voices resistance to this "merely utilitarian view." He raises the issue of the peculiarity of human experimentation quite independent of the question of possible injury to the subject. According to him, the wrong involved with making a person an experimental subject is not so much that we make him thereby a means to an end, since that happens in social contexts of all kinds, but that we make him a thing. He accuses us of reducing the person in human experimentation to a passive thing or token, or "sample" merely to be acted on.[24] This penetrating argument can assist researchers to structure the ethical issues in their deliberations of means and ends, the individual good and the common good, the private and the public welfare, all of which must be considered in informed consent.

Ideally, informed consent can be thought of as a collaborative endeavor involving truth telling on the part of the researcher and free choice on the part of the subject within a context of some degree of uncertainty. If we already knew all the possible risks and benefits of a given procedure or drug, then we would not need to undertake the research. In determining the most accurate risk-benefit ratio, we need a thoughtful, humane, and best-educated opinion. It may prove easier to detail these possibilities more adequately in research that has been tested on nonhuman subjects. It also may be more difficult to ascertain the psychologic impact or risks in all research. In addition, social science research may present special problems, since prior research on animals in most cases is inappropriate and impossible and the possible psychologic trauma experienced by human subjects sometimes remains underestimated and often unknown.

The Declaration of Helsinki says that research involving human subjects cannot legitimately be carried out unless the importance of the objective is in proportion to the inherent risk to the subject. Such inherent risks may be easier to measure and weigh in the risk-benefit calculus with biomedical research focused on physical aspects than with research focused on psychologic or social aspects. Nevertheless the Helsinki Declaration does say that every precaution should be taken to minimize the impact of the study on the subject's physical and mental integrity and on the personality of the subject.

It has been documented that the social sciences differ from the natural sciences in some fundamental ways. Although uncertainty exists in the natural sciences, the difficulty in observing and analyzing social reality presents other very complex social science problems. The objects of social science research are living, conditions, institutions, or human attitudes that combine changeability and rigidity in an unstable, and to some extent, and inscrutable pattern. Some social scientists have attempted to emulate the methods of natural sciences and this has led to a dangerous superficiality in approach at times. Such an analysis, regarded as strict or rigorous by natural science standards, may in social science research be lacking in both logical consistency and adequate reflection of reality.[25]

In the research projects of both natural science and social science, the importance of the research also becomes a factor. Some research may have minimum risk but also minimum benefits to the subject and/or society. Should such research be done? How could we either support it or not on moral grounds? If such research includes inconveniences, rather than risks to the human subjects, are there ethical considerations nonetheless? A more serious problem arises in the instance in which there is possible risk but minimum benefit involved in the study. In some research the procedure is so intrusive that the possible risks become more obvious, whereas when the procedures are less intrusive the possible risks may be overlooked. In each experimental situation such dimensions of the risk–benefit ratio need reviewing with the potential human subject before obtaining an informed consent.

In all research the possible dilemma arises as to the extent of the disclosure necessary to obtain a truly informed consent. When a patient engaged a physician or entered a hospital in the past, these actions in and of themselves often served as a blanket consent to such treatment as the physician or hospital staff, in the exercise of their professional judgment, deemed proper. Now the extent and the content of the disclosure for treatment purposes has expanded taking into account the patient's rights and the professional's obligations.

The similar problem in research, noted over 25 years ago, results from the combination of helplessness, lack of technical competence, and the emotional disturbance experienced in the sick role that make the patient a peculiarly vulnerable object for exploration.[26] This combined with the argument that patients do not want to know or can not understand has made informed consent a necessity. Patients not only have the right to know and to make decisions, but as one study found, the majority of them want to know what possible complications may be expected from any given procedure. This study concluded that the concern that informing the patient of possible complications will result in his refusal of the procedure is now outmoded.[27]

Baumrind has made one of the more profound observations in discussing the issue of human experimentation. She maintains that subjects are less adversely affected by physical pain or psychologic stress than by experiences that result in loss of trust in themselves and the investigators, and by extension in the meaningfulness of life itself. The researcher violates the fundamental moral principles of reciprocity and justice when he, using his position of trust, acts to deceive or degrade those whose extension of trust has been granted on the basis of a contrary role expectation. He behaves unjustly when he uses naive (trusting) subjects and then exploits their naivete, no matter if the direct resulting harm is small. The harm becomes cumulative both to the individual and to society.[28] This ethical position has had an impact on studies that, in the past, relied on deception in order to obtain their findings. Studies undertaken by Milgram, Rosenhand, and Hofling et al., provide but a few examples of such research.[29-31] Allison Lurie pushed the limits of deception in research and the undercover role of the scientist in her novel about two academic research sociologists.[32] Regardless of the importance of the findings in these and other such studies, a serious ethical dilemma underpins the entire research structure. To rely on deception means that the researcher totally violates the ethical principle of truthtelling and dupes the subject who cannot give his informed consent in a situation where he has not been told the real nature of the research or indeed that he is participating in research at all. This point usually raises the question as to whether this means that some research cannot or should not be done. Yes, it does possibly mean just that. Another question raised has to do with the problem of biasing the research by telling the subject too much detail. At least two solutions to the issue of informed consent in this case exist. First, it may be possible to redesign the research so that disclosure will not bias the study. Second, it may be possible to tell the subject some details and also discuss the fact that to go into more details would make the research findings less reliable. The latter solution has possible problems since, although the subject knows information is being withheld, he is not aware of the nature of the information.

As imperfect as it may be, the informed consent written procedure does accord the patient the status of a person, not an experimental animal, and provides a degree of assurance that he is being considered as an end, not merely a means. Respect for human dignity and individuality shares an historical comradeship with the freedom of scientific inquiry that is equally precious to modern liberalism. Like most norms, the basic principles of human experimentation have been formulated on such an abstract level that they provide only general guides to actual behavior. In so far as every treatment procedure and every involvement in research carries with them potential risk, it must be the patient or his guardian who has the right to decide not only whether to participate but also what factors are or are not relevant to his consent. This ethical position draws the line at full disclosure in most, if not all, instances, but also allows room for judgments to be made in the individual, concrete situation.[33] In the long run, all the regulations, reviews, and informed consent forms will serve a limited function unless the clinician and researcher bring their ethical reasoning and integrity to bear on these complex issues.[34–43]

INFORMED CONSENT AND SELECTED HUMAN SUBJECTS

The concept of informed consent rests on the assumption that the researcher will adequately inform the potential research subject, in language he can understand, so that the individual or his guardian will in fact understand the risks and benefits and will be in a position either to agree to participate or refuse to do so without negatively affecting his relationship with the researcher or the institution providing the service. Certain groups present special ethical problems and raise questions regarding the adequacy of informed consent. Research using students, prisoners, minors, the mentally ill, the mentally retarded, the elderly, especially those in an institution, and fetuses can and do raise many ethical dilemmas.

The problem of restricted choice can arise in a number of situations ranging from research with students to that with prisoners and other institutionalized persons. For example, when the instructor in a classroom asks the students to volunteer for research purposes, there exists at least the implied threat of loss of affection and possible decreased academic grades if the student does not volunteer. This becomes a situation of restricted choice for the student with ethical dilemmas involved. Previously, some institutions granted students credit for participating in research. This procedure raised the issue of infringement of the rights of those who did not volunteer or were not chosen after volunteering.[44]

A more serious ethical dilemma can occur in research using prisoners as human subjects. A number of individuals and groups have voiced concern about using prisoners in human experimentation.[44-54] These concerns have centered on a number of topics including behavioral research, behavior contol, drug tests, operant conditioning, psychosurgery, and castration, but the underlying ethical dilemma is to what extent can prisoners exercise freedom of choice in giving consent or refusing it. The issues of restrictive choice and possible coercion have been weighed against the benefits to the individual prisoner, usually remuneration and better living conditions for research subjects, reduced sentences in the past, benefits to society, and the obligations, if any, that the prisoner has to society. Many people concerned with this area of human experimentation believe that it may not be possible to overcome the serious ethical dilemmas. The fundamental ethical concepts embodied in the informed consent process can easily be violated in these circumstances.

With the mentally ill, a similar situation arises with the committed patient and the same ethical concerns may lead to the conclusion that informed consent is not a possibility. With the voluntary patients in institutions, informed consent may be an adequate safeguard because of his legal status; however, that status can change and his choices become restricted. Moreover, in either case, the patient's mental status due to his illness or to drugs and his ability to give consent must be viewed as the basis for a potential ethical dilemma.

Thus, to the mentally retarded, the problems are mental status, being institutionalized and dependent, and who speaks for and safeguards the rights of this individual being asked to serve as a human subject. If someone else consents for him, then that person must be informed and give consent with the best interest of the potential subject as the grounds for his actions. One can attempt to evaluate such action by asking what any reasonable person would do under the circumstances of making this decision. Most likely the characteristics of the ideal observer would be helpful in making the decision (see Chapter 2). Having all the information available, understanding potential consequences, coupled with the ability to visualize the experience as if it were happening to him, the observer, but also having the ability to be impartial, this observer ideally can make the best morally based decision. This observer represents an ideal, and not necessarily a reality, in any given individual; however, such characteristics may be found dispersed in a small group as they discuss the decision before them regarding risks and direct or indirect benefit, or the lack of them, to the subject.

Some doubts can be raised about the moral motivation of some parents in giving consent for their retarded institutionalized child to be part of a research study. This does not mean that all such parents are morally suspect, but a possible conflict of interest does exist in the situation. Possibly the child has been institutionalized because his parents reject him. In this case, conflict of interest looms larger than in a situation where the child has been placed in an institution because he cannot be physically managed at home or elsewhere.

The staff who conduct research with the mentally retarded in such an institution may have more of a conflict than some other researchers. Any research with the mentally retarded in any setting raises conflict of interest and other ethical dilemmas. A modified version of Rawls' publicity concept, mentioned in Chapter 2, provides one mechanism in dealing with this situation. A group, such as a ward unit group or a research review committee can examine the moral dimensions in a research protocol and determine whether the individuals being sought as human subjects should participate in the research and, if so, on what grounds taking into account their rights exercised in a situation of choice.

Some of the same issues come into play in research with minors.[55-60] An unwritten rule in many hospitals says that a child of seven or older can and should give his own informed consent, whereas a younger child has not developed moral reasoning and it falls to his parent or guardian to give consent. One of the most serious questions with any group, and especially vulnerable ones, including well children, involves research that is nontherapeutic or nonbeneficial to the subject. On what ethical grounds should research be conducted using either well children or mentally ill or retarded children where risks must be weighed against benefits. For normal children the benefits will be neither direct nor immediate in any tangible way. The questions become: should physically well, normal children ever be human subjects? If so, on what moral grounds? Should mentally ill or retarded children participate in any research and, if so, should it only be research that can potentially benefit them directly? If other research is to be permitted, on what moral grounds would these children become human subjects and who will speak for them in the informed consent procedure?

One area that has aroused much debate, that of fetal research, has also raised the issue of possible medical benefits gained as measured against the possible ethical costs of such research to society.[61-72] Some of this impassioned debate surrounding fetal research is tied to the different moral positions that people have taken on abortion. A discussion of the rights of the fetus can be found in Chapter 6.

The elderly, and particularly those in institutions such as nursing homes, represent another vulnerable group in the human subjects controversy. Essentially, many of the same issues mentioned above arise with this group. And as with some of the other groups, we tend to have negative attitudes toward the elderly that may blur some of the ethical considerations.[73-76]

One researcher, in writing about the inequitable allocation of research risks, makes the point that new knowledge designed to benefit all society must not be gained at the expense of any individual or any segment of society. To this end he would restrict experimentation to those research projects directly concerned with issues of the group of individuals used or research that has higher than average probability of benefiting the specific category of persons or would lead to such knowledge that could be expected to reduce the need for hospitalization or confinement.[77]

As with all potential human subjects for research projects, and certainly with these special problem groups, many ethical dilemmas emerge. Although some think that the goal of having human subjects spontaneously volunteer rather than being conscripted cannot be achieved, nevertheless, most believe that efforts to promote educated, informed consent are in order.[78,79] This effort to educate and inform should reach everyone including these groups and others such as the poor who depend more on public facilities where more training of health care personnel and more research probably occurs than in the private sector of the health care delivery system.

RISKS AND COMPENSATION

The individual's right to refuse to participate in research must be balanced against his obligations to society, the extent to which it will benefit him and/or others, and the potential risk involved. One 1976 report from the Department of Health, Education and Welfare, in an attempt to determine how many persons may be harmed by their participation in federally funded medical research, obtained data from 331 telephone interviews with investigators who conducted research in the preceding three years. A total of 133,000 human subjects participated in these studies. About half of the investigators reported that they did nontherapeutic research not expected to benefit study participants. Of about 93,000 subjects who participated in this nontherapeutic research, 0.8 percent were reported injured as a result of their participation.

The authors concluded that this injury rate compared to the annual rate of accidental injuries in this country that occur through ordinary living. Therefore the risks of participation in nontherapeutic research may be no greater than those of everyday life. Of the 39,000 or so individuals who participated in therapeutic research in which treatments that could be expected to benefit the participants who were involved, 10.8 percent were reported as being injured in some way. Again, however, this rate compares to that experienced as a result of ordinary treatment outside the research setting.[80]

The topic of compensating injured research subjects has received attention both from the law and from ethicists.[81-83] The ethicist James Childress has developed a detailed moral argument to use in thinking through the ethical dilemmas of this issue.[84] He considers the basis, scope, and limits of society's obligations to compensate injured research subjects within the framework of justice. Reparative justice, rendering each person his or her due, focuses on the fault of one party for an injury to another party, and the party causing the injury is blameworthy and held liable for it. On the other hand, compensatory justice is giving a person his or her due by taking account of a previous state of affairs and attempting to restore a "fallen" individual or group to it. Restoration can rarely be literal, and therefore it most often requires a monetary substitute. According to Childress, compensatory justice is a concrete application of the principle of fairness in the imposition of risks for the benefit of society. From this moral argument, only briefly touched upon here, he draws the conclusion that informed consent does not constitute a waiver of claims for compensation.

Informed consent implies joint adventurers in a common cause, a partnership between subject and investigator, or a process of coinvestigation. It is the propensity to overreach this joint adventure, even in a good cause, that makes consent necessary. However, this agreement can be no substitute for the wisdom and moral integrity of the researcher.[85-86]

INFORMED CONSENT AND NURSING

In the most fundamental sense, the moral principle at stake in informed consent was addressed by Kant when he said that we ought to treat mankind as an end, and never merely as a means.[87] But, as has been noted, it sounds strange to speak of persons as ends even though the Kantian formula is familiar to us. As has been implied so far in this chapter, as well as in other chapters, we regard persons as valuable in themselves, not for what we can get out of them but because they are persons. To say that something, in this case, persons, is valuable in itself does not exclude the possibility that it is also valuable as a means. Many of our problems arise when we consider persons *merely* as a means. The moral principle therefore is that we ought to treat people as valuable in themselves and not only as useful instruments.[88]

A number of comments have been made about ethical issues or dilemmas and human rights as related to nursing practice and research.[89-92] This present discussion includes selected papers that have pioneered in this topic as it affects nursing. Abdellah, in a paper based on a presentation at the 1967 National League for Nursing Convention, noted that as nursing research focused more on clinical problems, the legal and ethical aspects would become more apparent. Although clinical nursing research may differ from medical research in the extent and kind of risk to patients, nevertheless, many similar problems exist in both disciplines in their conduct of research. At that time, according to Abdellah, much, if not most, clinical nursing research used the behavioral science methods such as interviews, questionnaires, and observations to obtain data. Ethical issues involved a number of factors including the right to privacy or to withhold information. It is helpful to know that just two years before, in June 1965, the United States Supreme Court had given an opinion to the case of *Griswold et al.* v. *Connecticut,* which dealt with an alledged infringement of the right of privacy in marriage. In so doing, the Court established that, although privacy was not guaranteed in so many words by the Constitution or the Bill of Rights, it was a basic and fundamental right deeply rooted in our society. Mr. Justice Douglas delivered the opinion of the Court and discussed the idea that various other guarantees in the Constitution created zones of individual privacy.[93]

Nurse investigators in the mid-1960s were just beginning to make inroads in biologic research. Among other problems, the use of double-blind techniques requiring the withholding of certain treatment information from both the patient and the staff caring for the patient necessitates skilled handling to protect the subject. Such a situation requires value judgments grounded in professional ethics to determine the degree of risk compared with the potential benefits obtained. At that time, the nature of consent to participate in research as a human subject could be implicit, explicit, or a written statement since the fact that the patient was admitted to a hospital implied a certain degree of implicit consent.[94] With the advent of governmental guidelines for the use of human subjects and the establishment of peer review committees to assist in safeguarding the rights of human subjects through a formal informed consent procedure, the informal and blanket mechanisms, which could be too easily abused, became ancient history.

In 1969, Berthold wrote a detailed paper based on a review of the literature and focused on the larger topic of maintaining human rights and values in the midst of a scientific–technologic revolution and the concomitant social revolution. She developed the idea that the right of the individual in American society to dignity, self-respect, and freedom for self-determination has been in conflict with the rights and long-range interests of society on many occasions and on various issues. Berthold goes on to say that these conflicts have generally been characterized as involving humanitarian, libertarian, and scientific values. Humanitarian values have to do with respect for the sanctity of human life and the safeguards needed to protect the subject from physical or emotional harm. Libertarian values have to do with the individual's political, civil, and individual rights to self-respect, dignity, freedom of thought and action, and the safeguards needed to protect the individual from invasion of his privacy without his knowledge and consent. Scientific values have to do with the extension of knowledge for knowledge's sake and the safeguards needed to protect the right to know anything that may be known or discovered about any part of the universe. These different values lead to competing moral claims in specific situations that must be balanced against one another within the process of moral reasoning.[95]

Scientific inquiry can involve several specific ethical issues, all of which should be considered by the nurse investigator when designing the research as well as by the potential human subject prior to giving informed consent. These issues include: (1) loss of dignity and autonomy, (2) invasion of privacy, (3) time and/or energy requirement, (4) mental and physical discomfort or pain, and (5) risk of physical or emotional injury. These must be weighed against potential benefits for the subject himself, for people like him, e.g., diabetics, and for the general good of all people.

In 1970, Batey raised the question as to when and to what extent does the issue of the rights of human subjects become a methodologic issue in nursing research. She made the point that researchers have historically been accorded considerable prestige; however, now less and less people respond compliantly and with unquestioning deference to others who hold prestigious positions. She also asks whether there is a metaprofessional ethic or a set of values guiding nurse researchers, not the conduct of inquiry, but in the context in which it is carried out. Additionally, do nurse researchers share a set of values directed toward optimizing the conditions requisite to the fulfillment of the aims of science?[96]

The American Nurses' Association has been active in developing guidelines on ethical values for the nurse in research. In 1968 the Committee on Research and Studies said that nursing was committed to the identification and elaboration of a body of scientific knowledge specific to nursing represented by the descriptive, explanatory, and predictive principles that guide nursing practice for the provision of optimal nursing services to society. The Association reaffirmed its belief in the rights and the responsibilities of members of the profession to conduct research and to meet its obligations to those members by establishing guidelines on ethical values. In discussing these ethical dimensions within the framework of protecting human rights, the Association elaborated on the rights to privacy, to self-determination, to conservation of personal resources, to freedom from arbitrary hurt, and to freedom from intrinsic risk of injury. The rights of minors and incompetent persons, such as young children or unconscious patients, as well as the informed consent process were also discussed. Essentially, the Association's position rests on the idea that the relationship of trust between subject and investigator requires that the subject be assured that he will be treated fairly; and that no discomfort, risk, or inconvenience, beyond that initially stated in obtaining informed consent, will be imposed without further permission being obtained from the subject.[97]

With this preliminary work on guidelines serving as a background, the Association acknowledged the changes that had occurred in the early 1970s in the area of research regulations and guidelines for informed consent by publishing the position paper on human rights developed by the Commission on Nursing Research.[98] One very important aspect of this document is its statement on human rights for the nurse:

Whenever nurses perform activities that are components of clinical research (whether directed by physicians, nurses, or other investigators) the need for protection of human rights must extend to the practitioners who are expected to participate in new and untried practices as well as subjects who are recipients of them. The concept of informed consent applies not only to subjects *per se* but also to any workers who are expected as part of their daily work to implement activities that are potentially or actually carry risk for others or have uncertain outcomes.

Implementation of this guideline implies the need for written statements about conditions of employment and any special expectations about work performance above and beyond that usually expected of a person occupying the position of nurse. In advance of such employment, nurses need to know if they will be expected to provide medicines, treatments, and other procedures as part of double-blind investigations. They need to know in advance if the work requires them to function as data collectors for research in addition to their role as nurses engaged in the delivery of patient care services. Conditions of employment must also provide for the option of not participating in clinical research if these work expectations are not spelled out in advance of employment.[99]

The nurse who conducts research does not differ from her colleagues in other disciplines. Her research protocol and activities must insure that the human subject will be informed in understandable language and will in no way be coerced to participate or continue in the study, but will be free to experience his freedom of self-determination. As stated previously, essentially only the integrity and the ethics of the investigator will safeguard the safety and the rights of the human subject. The patient's safety and his rights must be attended to within the context of the advancement of nursing knowledge, the growing number of nurses engaged in an academic and/or a research career, and the rising professionalism of nursing. These factors can act to either enhance or inhibit a fuller discussion within the profession of the issues involved in research with human subjects, informed consent, and the conflicting moral claims which create ethical dilemmas for the nurse researcher who is the principle investigator and for the nurse in the clinical setting who assists in another's research.

REFERENCES

1. Fallows J: Lo, the poor animals. Atlantic Monthly, September 1976, pp 58–65
2. Bernard C: An Introduction to the Study of Experimental Medicine. New York, Macmillan, 1927
3. Fortner v Koch, 272 Mich 273, 282, 261, N.W. 1935
4. Vaux K: Biomedical Ethics. New York, Harper & Row, 1974, pp 29–30
5. Katz J: The education of the physician investigator. Daedalus 98: 480–83, 1969
6. Sessoms SM: Investigational drugs: guiding principles in medical research involving humans. Hospitals, January, 1958, pp 44–47
7. US Department of Health, Education and Welfare: Grants Administration Manual, Washington, DC, 1971
8. Langer E: Human experimentation: New York verdict affirms patients' rights. Science, February 1966, pp 663–66
9. Krugman S, Giles JP: Viral hepatitis: new light on an old disease. JAMA, May 11, 1970, pp. 1019–21
10. US Public Health Service, Final Report of the Tuskegee Syphilis Study Ad Hoc Advisory Panel. Washington, DC, 1973
11. Ad Hoc Subcommittee on Use of Human Subjects in Safety Evaluation: Some Considerations in the Use of Human Subjects in Safety Evaluation of Pesticides and Food Chemicals. Washington, DC, National Academy of Sciences, 1965
12. Culliton BJ: Policy issues in the federal support of biomedical research: a review. Public Sci, March 1974, pp 5–10
13. Frankel MS: The development of policy guidelines governing human experimentation in the United States. Ethics Sci Med, May 1975, pp 43–59

14. Gray BH: An assessment of institutional review committees in human experimentation. Med Care, April 1975, pp 318-28
15. Human experimentation: the regulation controversy. Society, November/December 1975, pp 4-12
16. US, Congress, Senate, Subcommittee on Health: Federal Regulations of Human Experimentation. 93rd Congr, 1st sess, May 1975
17. US Department of Health, Education and Welfare, National Institutes of Health: Protection of human subjects. Federal Register 39, May 30, 1974, Pt 2
18. Veatch RM: Human experimentation committees: professional or representative? Hastings Cent Rep, October 1975, pp 31-40
19. Curran WJ: Current legal issues in clinical investigation with particular attention to the balance between the rights of the individual and the needs of society. Proceedings of the Sixth Annual Meeting of the American College of Neuropsychopharmacology, San Juan, Puerto Rico. December 12-15, 1967, pp 337-43
20. Beecher HK: Ethics and clinical research. New Engl J Med, June 16, 1966, pp 1354-60
21. Barber B: The ethics of experimentation with human subjects. Scientific American, February 1976, pp 25-31
22. Gray BH: Human Subjects in Medical Experimentation. New York, Wiley, 1975
23. McDermott W: Opening comments: a colloquium on ethical dilemmas from medical advances. Ann Int Med, September 1967, pp 39-42
24. Jonas H: Philosophical reflections on experimenting with human subjects. In Freund PA (ed): Experimentation with Human Subjects, Braziller, 1969, pp 1-31
25. Myrdal G: Biases in social research. In Tiselius A, Nilsson S (eds): The Place of Value in a World of Fact. New York, Wiley, 1970, p 156
26. Parsons T: The Social System. Glencoe, Ill, Free Press, 1951, p 437
27. Alfidi RJ: Informed consent—a study of patient reaction. JAMA, May 24, 1971, pp 1325-29
28. Baumrind D: Principles of ethical conduct in the treatment of subjects. Am Psychol, October 1971, pp 887-96
29. Milgram S: Some conditions of obedience and disobedience to authority. Human Relations, February, 1965, pp 57-75
30. Rosenhand DL: On being sane in insane places. Science, January 19, 1973, pp 250-58
31. Hofling C, Brotzman E, Dalrymple S, Graves N, Pierce CM: An experimental study in nurse–patient relationships. J Nerv Ment Dis 113:171-80, 1966
32. Lurie A: Imaginary Friends. New York, Avon, 1975
33. Brody EB: The right to know. J Nerv Ment Dis 161:73-81, 1971
34. Barber B, Lally JJ, Makarushka JL, Sullivan D: Research on Human Subjects: Problems of Social Control in Medical Experimentation. New York, Russell Sage, 1973

35. Beecher HK: Research and the Individual: Human Studies. Boston, Little, Brown, 1970

36. National Academy of Sciences: Experimentation and Research with Humans: Values in Conflict. Washington, DC, The Academy, 1975

37. Lally JJ, Barber B: The compassionate physician: frequency and social determinants of physician-investigator concern for human subjects. Social Forces, December 1974, p 289-96

38. Lasagna L: The Conflict of Interest between Physician as Therapist and Experimenter. Philadelphia, Society for Health and Human Values, 1975

39. Spiro HM: Constraint and consent—on being a patient and a subject. New Engl J Med, November 27, 1975, pp 1134-35

40. Visscher MB: Ethical Constraints and Imperatives in Medical Research. Springfield, Ill, Thomas, 1975

41. Mills DH: Whither informed consent? JAMA, July 15, 1974, pp 305-10

42. Kelman HC: A Time to Speak: On Human Values and Social Research. San Francisco, Jossey-Bass, 1968

43. Warwick DP: Tearoom trade: means and ends in social research. Hastings Cent Stud, 1:27-38, 1973

44. Lasagna L: Special subjects in human experimentation. Daedalus 98: 456-57, 1969

45. McDonald JC: Why prisoners volunteer to be experimental subjects. JAMA, November 6, 1967, pp 175-76

46. Hodges RE, Bean WB: The use of prisoners for medical research. JAMA, November 6, 1967, pp 177-79

47. Ayd FJ: Drug studies in prisoner volunteers. South Med J, April, 1972, pp 440-44

48. Capron AM: Medical research in prisons. Hastings Cent Rep, June, 1973, pp 4-6

49. Mitford J: Experimentation behind bars. Atlantic Monthly, January, 1973, pp 64-73

50. Jonsen AR et al: Biomedical Experimentation on Prisoners: Review of Practices and Problems and Proposal of a New Regulatory Approach. San Francisco, University of California School of Medicine, Health Policy Program, September 1975

51. Burt RA: Why we should keep prisoners from the doctors: reflections on the Detroit psychosurgery case. Hastings Cent Rep, February 1975, pp 25-34

52. Klerman G, Dworkin G: Case studies in bioethics: can convicts consent to castration? Hastings Cent Rep, October 1975, pp 17-19

53. Rubin JS: Breaking into the prison: conducting a medical research project. Am J Psychiatr, February 1976, pp 230-32

54. Wolstenholme GEW, O'Connor M: Medical Care of Prisoners and Detainees. New York, Elsevier, 1973

55. Curran WJ, Beecher HK: Experimentation in children. JAMA, October 6, 1969, pp 77-83

56. Ramsey P: The Patient as Person. New Haven, Yale University Press, 1970, pp 1–58

57. Schwartz AH: Children's concepts of research hospitalization. New Engl J Med, September 21, 1972, pp 589–92

58. McCormick RA: Proxy consent in the experimentation situation. Perspect Biol Med, Autumn 1974, pp 2–20

59. Lower CU et al: Nontherapeutic research on children: an ethical dilemma. J. Pediatr, April, 1974, pp 468–73

60. Campbell AGM: Infants, children and informed consent. Br Med J, August 3, 1974, pp 334–38

61. Ayd FJ Jr: Fetology: medical and ethical implications of intervention in the prenatal period. Ann NY Acad Sci 169:376–81, 1970

62. Kass L: Babies by means of in vitro fertilization: unethical experiments on the unborn? New Engl J Med, November 18, 1971, pp 1174–78

63. Reback GL: Fetal experimentation: moral, legal, and medical implications. Stanford Law Review, May 1974, pp 1191–207

64. Fost N: Our curious attitudes toward the fetus. Hastings Cent Rep, February 1974, pp 4–5

65. Dykes MHM, Czapek EE: Regulations and legislation concerning abortus research. JAMA, September 2, 1974, pp 1303–4

66. Curran WJ: Experimentation becomes a crime: fetal research in Massachusetts. New Engl J Med, February 6, 1975, pp 300–301

67. Gaylin W, Lappé M: Fetal politics: the debate on experimenting with the unborn. Atlantic Monthly, May 1975, pp 66–73

68. Hart DS: Fetal research and antiabortion politics; holding science hostage. Family Plan Perspect, March–April 1975, pp 72–82

69. Lappé M: The moral claims of the wanted fetus. Hastings Cent Rep, April 1975, pp 11–14

70. Powledge TM: Fetal experimentation: sorting out the issues. Hastings Cent Rep, April 1975, pp 8–10

71. Ramsey P: The Ethics of Fetal Research. New Haven, Yale University Press, 1975

72. Tiefel HO: The cost of fetal research: ethical considerations. New Engl J Med, January 8, 1976, pp 85–90

73. Mendelson MA: Tender Loving Greed. New York, Knopf, 1974

74. Hess BB: Stereotypes of the aged. J Commun Autumn, 1974, pp 76–85

75. Kaplan J: In search of policies for card of the aged. In Tancredi LR: Ethics of Health Care. Washington, DC, National Academy of Sciences, 1974

76. Butler RN: Why Survive? Being Old in America. New York, Harper & Row, 1975

77. Marston RQ: Research on minors, prisoners and the mentally ill. New Engl J Med, January 18, 1973, pp 158–59

78. Jonas H: op cit

79. Ingelfinger FJ: Informed (but uneducated) consent. New Engl J Med, August 31, 1972, pp 465–66
80. Brody JE: Study finds injury risk in medical research similar to normal living. New York Times, September 19, 1976, p 54
81. Medical experiment insurance. Columbia Law Review, May 1970, p 974
82. Morris N: Compensation and the Good Samaritan. In Ratcliffe JM: The Good Samaritan and the Law. Garden City, NJ, Doubleday, 1966, p 136
83. Adams BR, Shea-Stonum M: Toward a theory of control of medical experimentation with human subjects: the role of compensation. Case Wester Reserve Law Review, Spring 1975, p 637
84. Childress JF: Compensating injured research subjects: the moral arguments. Hastings Cent Rep, December 1976, pp 21–27
85. Ramsey P: op cit, pp 6–8
86. Katz J: Experimentation with Human Beings. New York, Russell Sage 1972
87. Kant I: The Fundamental Principles of the Metaphysics of Morals. London, Hutchinson's University Library, 1948
88. Downie RS, Telfer E: Respect for Persons. New York, Schocken Books, 1970, pp 14–15
89. Marietta DE Jr: On using people. Ethics, April 1972, pp 232–38
90. Carpenter WT: The nurse's role in informed consent. Nurs Times, July 3, 1975, pp 1049–51
91. Hubbard S, DeVita V: Chemotherapy research: the nurse in oncology. Am J Nurs, April 1976, pp 560–65
92. Jacobson SF: Ethical issues in experimentation with human subjects. Nurs Forum 12 (1): 58–71, 1973
93. Abdellah FG: Approaches to protecting the rights of human subjects. Nurs Res, Fall 1967, pp 316–20
94. Griswold et al v. Connecticut, 381 U.S. 479 (1965)
95. Berthold JS: Advancement of science and technology while maintaining human rights and values. Nurs Res, November–December 1969, pp 514–22
96. Batey MV: Some methodological issues in research. Nurs Res, November–December 1970, pp 511–16
97. ANA Committee on Research and Studies: The nurse in research: ANA guidelines on ethical values. Nurs Res, March–April 1968, pp 104–7
98. ANA Commission on Nursing Research: Human Rights Guidelines for Nurses in Clinical and Other Research. Kansas City, ANA, 1975
99. Ibid: pp 3–4

6

ABORTION

ABORTION AND BIRTH CONTROL

Abortion, the expulsion or removal of the products of conception from the uterus, generally occurs before the 28th week of pregnancy. Spontaneous abortion occurs as a result of a variety of endogenous and exogenous causes, excluding intentional human interference. Such human interference, called induced abortion, to deliberately terminate a pregnancy, performed either legally or illegally, relies on a number of different methods.[1] The method used depends, in part, on timing or how long the pregnancy has existed. Medically speaking, abortion during the first trimester is easiest to perform and safest for the woman involved. However, women do undergo abortion during the second trimester or until the fetus becomes viable. Viability of the fetus means that is has potential ability to live outside the uterus, albeit with artificial means if necessary.[2] Uncertainty surrounds the notion of just when viability occurs and definitions vary from 20 to 24 weeks. In the last trimester, abortion presents increased dangers to the woman and the likelihood of delivering a live fetus also increases.

Statistically speaking, abortion, one of the world's oldest and most popular methods of birth control, if performed under good conditions early in pregnancy, has become as safe as or safer than carrying a baby to full term.[3] The argument can be made that other effective methods of contraception have been developed that could replace abortion in most cases as a means of birth control. Furthermore, these alternatives to abortion have the potential of presenting fewer ethical dilemmas for many who use them. However, several factors must be taken into account before pursuing this line of argument very far. First, not all people receive sound knowledge about sex and reproduction and in many places people still continue to do battle over sex education in the schools. Second, research findings have begun to throw into question the safety of the most effective birth control device, the pill. And finally, the fact remains that people do not necessarily act on information and knowledge they have even when the results of their actions may prove detrimental to their health or lives. For example, smoking, driving while intoxicated, and having sexual intercourse without using some form of contraception when the couple does not want a pregnancy all support this fact. Such devices succeed in preventing unwanted pregnancies only if used consistently. The nature of human sexuality and the complex motivations that people bring to their sexual experiences lend themselves to mishaps. For these and other reasons not discussed here, abortion as a form of birth control remains with us.

BACKGROUND

Inevitably, the statistical data on legal or illegal abortions performed in the past cannot be stated with certainty. One study of legal abortion covering the years 1957 through 1962 indicated that the women questioned had 1039 abortions as against 522,600 live births. This means there existed a ratio of about two abortions to every 1000 live births. Using this ratio and extrapolating it to about four million yearly deliveries in this country, we could make an educated guess that, for the years of the study, approximately 8000 legal abortions were performed annually.[4] We have, for obvious reasons, even fewer facts about illegal abortions. However, some observations have been made that suggest certain patterns and concerns. In the United States prior to the 1973 Supreme Court decision, abortion had been largely performed clandestinely by physicians, especially for the financially well off. The poor had been more likely to abort themselves or to resort to nonmedical amateurs. The majority of those aborted had been married women with several children. As an aftermath of illegal abortion, death and invalidism have not been inconsiderable. In the 1960s, almost 50 percent of deaths in New York City associated with pregnancy and birth resulted from illegal abortions.[5] The death rate from abortion in Hungary, where women can easily obtain a legal abortion, has been reported as less than six per 100,000. In the United States, the death rate resulting from the removal of tonsils and adenoids has been put at 17 per 100,000, while the death rate from childbirth and its complications has been reported as 24 per 100,000.[6] The past 35 years have seen a downward trend in both reported maternal mortality, excluding abortion, and in reported mortality from abortion as well. These declines primarily reflect progress in the prevention and treatment of puerperal infection and other complications associated with pregnancy and childbirth. In these years of declining mortality rates, mortality from abortion in the United States remained much higher among nonwhite women than among white women.[7]

Numerous regional and national studies conducted during the last 20 years indicate that the poor, the less educated, and blacks want about the same number of children as others in this society.[8-12] Despite the desire for relatively small families, the studies also show that these groups tend to have larger families than they want. At every point of choice, the middle- and upper-class white woman has tended to have greater access to contraception, abortion, forced marriage, and adoption. Prior to the 1973 abortion law, research data, collected in those states where repeal laws had been passed, demonstrated that when abortion became more readily available, the lower socioeconomic groups made the greatest use of abortion facilities.[13-16]

One of the reasons given in the past for not making abortions accessible has been the psychiatric concern that such a traumatic procedure would lead to a burden of guilt and possibly to mental illness. Such statements rarely could be supported by reliable scientific evidence involving a large sample. According to one psychiatrist, a careful review of the literature reveals that little justification for this traditional opinion exists.[17] Another psychiatrist refers to the myth of serious emotional sequelae, but goes on to say that even psychiatric illness is no reason to deny a woman an abortion. In his experience most normal women respond to abortion with mild feelings of depression without serious aftereffects, while mentally ill women respond with improved mental attitudes.[18] Both the social and psychologic dimensions of abortion require further study. These dimensions interact with the general attitudes toward abortion held by society, including those of health professionals.

Although change seems inevitable and rapid, attitudes do take time to shift on many important issues. Approximately seven national surveys, conducted between 1962 and 1969 on attitudes toward abortion, showed that public opinion changed very little during these eight years.[19] Although the abortion controversy came into sharp focus during the 1960s and the underlying issues had been with us for many years, not until 1972 did a survey show more favorable public attitudes toward abortion.[20] Although some physicians have favored the liberalized abortion laws, opposition to abortion has nevertheless remained widespread. Essentially, reluctance, if not opposition, reflects the attitude of many in the medical profession. The enormous influence of this segment of the profession on whether women find abortions difficult or easier to obtain becomes a critical favor.[21] Some recent data indicate that in 1976 approximately 700,000 women wanted abortions but were unable to obtain them. Furthermore, only 27 percent of all general non-Catholic hospitals in the country performed abortions.[22]

A number of other medical procedures influencing abortion as a birth control measure have been developed. Not without their own ethical and legal issues, sterilization and artificial insemination have received more publicity in recent years and may develop into viable alternatives for controlling population. Amniocentesis, the procedure whereby a sample of amniotic fluid can be obtained for analysis, may eventually become a routine part of good prenatal care. In the mid-1960s the shift in the focus of amniocentesis from a tool used in the latter stages of pregnancy to detect and treat abnormalities to a means of early detection and abortion began almost imperceptibly.[23] This change has been received with positive reactions by those who view the procedure as a means of treating abnormalities in utero or early detection and abortion of an abnormal fetus when treatment cannot be undertaken. Others, however, have raised the myriad of ethical dilemmas that surround the procedure. One writer puts it profoundly when he says that the lure of a genetic test for a normal and in the future an optimal infant threatens to reinforce a trend in our society toward typecasting the less-than-optimal into categories for assortment and ultimate disposal.[24]

A great many factors intersect in any discussion on abortion: medical, sociologic, psychologic, technologic, and the attitudes grounded in philosophical and moral concerns that the public has developed. This background information coupled with the overview of the historical and social context of abortion to follow will help us to understand more fully the ethical dilemmas surrounding abortion.

THE LARGER CONTEXTS

In 1973, the United States Supreme Court declared abortion a lawful act during the first trimester of pregnancy. After the first trimester, the state can restrict abortion through regulations protecting the pregnant woman's health. After viability, the state may regulate or forbid abortion except in those instances where medical judgments indicate its necessity to safeguard the health or life of the pregnant woman.[25,26] In arguing the first case, *Roe* v. *Wade*, before the Court, the lawyer traced the legal history of abortion. The restrictive criminal abortion laws in effect at the time the Court heard the case derived from statutory changes effected in the main during the latter half of the nineteenth century. A brief historical view of religious attitudes, the law, and scientific and social developments form the larger context within which to understand the Court's decision regarding abortion.

HISTORICAL CONTEXT

At the time of the Persian Empire, abortifacients were accessible and individuals who performed criminal abortions received severe punishment. In ancient Greece and during the Roman era people resorted to abortion without scruple.[27] Plato in *The Republic* and Aristotle in *Politics* described abortion as a means of preventing excess population. Neither Greek nor Roman law afforded protection to the unborn fetus. Furthermore, the religions practiced in these cultures did not bar abortion; however, philosophers, religious teachers, and physicians debated the morality of performing abortions. In this climate, the Hippocratic Oath developed and took a position against abortion. One theory explains this radical departure from the prevailing practice of the time in light of the Pythagorean dogma.[28] Most Greek thinkers, except for the Pythagorean school, commended abortion, at least prior to viability. For the Pythagoreans the embryo became animated or infused with a soul from the moment of conception so that abortion meant destroying a living being. The abortion clause in the Hippocratic Oath reflects Pythagorean doctrine, a small segment of Greek opinion at the time. Furthermore, medical writings down to Galen's time (130-200 A.D.) provided evidence of violation of almost every injunction of the oath. For example, Soranos (98-138 A.D.), a Greek from Ephesus, became Rome's leading gynecologist and in his writings he lists the reasons for abortion and the means to achieve it.[29] Only at the end of antiquity, with the emerging teachings of Christianity, which agreed with the Pythagorean ethic, did the Oath become the nucleus of all medical ethics and was regarded as the embodiment of truth. For some this historical context explains what appears to them as the rigidity of the Hippocratic Oath.

The Greco-Roman world, distinguished by its indifference to fetal life, also saw the development of Christianity, which gave rise to values in opposition and conflict with the generally held popular beliefs. The specific Christian teaching on abortion developed in a theological context of the Christian valuation of life grounded in the Old Testament command to love your neighbor as yourself (Lev. 19:18). The basis for fulfillment of this commandment, found in the New Testament, emphasized the sacrifice of man's life for another (John 15:13) embodied in the self-sacrifice of Jesus. Jesus commanded his disciples to love one another as he had loved them (John 15:32). From this commandment of love, the Christian valuation of life evolved.[30]

Abortion, as a subject of concern to secular humanists and theologians, has a long history. At the heart of this complex discourse lies the question of how do you determine the humanity of a being. The Catholic position on abortion has been clearly stated since the late 1880s and has been reaffirmed by recent Popes. Catholics, as well as some other religious leaders, believe the embryo becomes a human being with a soul from the moment of conception. Some of the early teachers of the Church, however, including St. Thomas Aquinas, did not consider it possible for an unformed embryo to have a soul and placed ensoulment at about three months after conception when the fetus had developed a recognizable human shape. Along with this concept of ensoulment, Catholics reject abortion on the grounds that unborn children needed baptism. Although not as strongly upheld in the Church today, this doctrine of baptizing the endangered fetus still holds. The official position of Catholic leaders today involves the concept of ensoulment that defines the fetus from conception as a human being and basically can be analyzed as a refusal to discriminate among human beings on the basis of the varying potentialities.

Protestant views vary due to the numerous sects and groups involved. Although many Protestants do not agree with the Catholic Church on ensoulment, they do regard abortion as undesirable, though not a mortal sin, since the embryo as an entity should be preserved from unnecessary destruction. Generally, for Protestants, the concept of the sacredness of life has served as an obstacle to the wanton and thoughtless performance of abortion. In attempting to determine when human life begins, most Protestant leaders agree that by the time of quickening, or the first recognizable movements of the fetus in utero, one can define the fetus as a human being.

One Protestant writer outlines pertinent principles that can be stipulated for reflection and reduces them to the following simplified scheme: First, life must be preserved rather than destroyed; second, protection must be provided especially to those who cannot assert their own right to life, and third, exceptions to these rules exist such as (a) medical indications that make therapeutic abortion morally viable, (b) the pregnancy resulted from a sexual crime, (c) the social and the emotional conditions do not appear beneficial for the well-being of the mother and child.[31] This writer replaces the determination of an action as right or wrong according to its conformity to a rule and its application by stressing the primacy of the person and human relationships along with the concreteness of the choice within limited possibilities. In the case of abortion, he maintains that no guarantee of an objectively right action can be given since several values, all objectively important, exist. Furthermore, these values do not resolve themselves into a harmonious relation to each other. Since there is not a single overriding determination of what constitutes a right action, there can be no unambiguously right act.[32]

Ancient Jewish writings consider the fetus a living being when it detaches itself from the mother. According to the Talmud this occurs when the head has emerged from the birth canal. Orthodox Jewish leaders maintain that abortion is morally wrong at any time, except when the mother's life becomes seriously threatened. Reform Jews would accept more reasons for abortion. For all practical purposes, the relatively permissive attitudes of Conservative and Reform Judaism can be equated with a growing number of Protestant sects on the topic of abortion.[33]

Briefly, Buddhists condemn killing of life but define commencement of life rather loosely whereas the Shinto religion recognizes the infant as a living being after birth. The Islamic religion takes the stance that abortion is permissible until the embryo develops into the human shape or for 120 days after conception.[34]

LEGAL CONTEXT

The legal aspects of abortion have been influenced by religious developments and definitions. In the fourth century A.D., the Roman Empire developed the first laws against abortion in a time when Christian influence began to be felt. However, in the common law, abortion performed prior to quickening, 16 to 18 weeks, was not an indictable offense.[35] This lack of a common-law crime for abortion occurring before quickening seems to have been influenced by theologic concepts, civil and canon law concepts, and philosophical concepts of the beginning of life, of when the embryo became infused with a soul. Christian theology and canon law fixed the point of animation at 40 days for a male and 80 days for a female, a view that persisted until the nineteenth century. General agreement developed that prior to animation, the fetus was part of the mother and therefore its destruction was not homicide. However, due to the uncertainty as to the exact time of animation and perhaps influenced by Aquinas' definition of movement in utero as one criterion of life, Bracton, in the first references to abortion in English criminal law, wrote in 1640 that to abort a woman is homicide if the embryo were formed and especially if it were animated.[36] Other English legal scholars, such as Edward Coke, Matthew Hale, and William Russell, used the concept of quickening to develop the common law precedents regarding abortion. In 1803 England's first criminal abortion statute made the abortion of a quick fetus a capital crime. This law also provided lesser penalties for the felony of abortion that occurred before quickening. In 1967, the British Parliament enacted a new, liberal abortion law.

In the United States, generally speaking, the law in effect until the middle of the nineteenth century was the pre-existing English common law. In the post-Civil War years legislation began to replace the common law. These final statutes were lenient with abortion before quickening, but dealt severely with abortion after quickening. During the middle and late nineteenth century, the quickening distinction disappeared from the statutory law in most states and the penalties for performing an abortion increased.[37] For approximately 100 years, the United States outlawed practically all abortions. Some states made slight changes in their abortion laws before 1959; however, the movement toward definite reform, pioneered by Colorado, and based on the American Law Institute's Model Penal Code, occurred in 1967. Rather than creating an abortion-mill situation as feared by its critics, this statute resulted in caution on the part of physicians and hospitals.[38]

The United States Supreme Court decision, delivered on January 22, 1973, in a seven to two decision, declared both an original statute (Texas, *Roe* v. *Wade*) and a reform statute (Georgia, *Doe* v. *Bolton*) unconstitutional. As stated earlier, the Court ruled that a state could not interfere in the abortion decision between a woman and her physician during the first trimester. In the second trimester, when abortion becomes more hazardous, the state's interest in the woman's health permits the enactment of regulation to protect maternal health. Beyond these procedural requirements, the abortion decision still rests with the woman and her physician. After the fetus reaches viability, or approximately the last trimester, the state can exercise its interest in promoting potential human life. At this stage, the state can prohibit abortion except when the necessity arises to preserve the life or health of the mother. The Court did not support the position that a woman has an absolute right to abortion regardless of circumstances; however, the position it did take made legal abortion potentially more available than at any time in the United States during the twentieth century. In 1976 the Court dealt with several additional issues regarding abortion, the consent of the spouse, the right of a minor to an abortion, and whether the state can stop a particular method of abortion.

The major grounds in the Court's decision evolved from the 14th Amendment of the Constitution and its concept of personal liberty and developed into the woman's right to privacy that, according to the Court, "is broad enough to encompass a woman's decision whether or not to terminate her pregnancy." As late as 1977, the pro-abortionists continued to fight to remove the remaining restriction in the abortion law, while the anti-abortionists strove for a Constitutional amendment that would recognize a fetus' right to life. In light of its long history and the great passions generated by the abortion issue, continuation of this controversy can be expected in and out of legislatures and courts. The abortion laws prior to 1973 express a responsibility ethic that has been an important aspect of the psychosocial structure in this society. In effect the laws have said that people are and must be responsible for the consequences of their acts; whether or not they are, they ought to be.[39]

In January 1977, Joseph Califano, then Health, Education and Welfare Secretary-designate, in a confirmation hearing before a Senate Committee said that he would oppose the use of federal funds for abortions. This is but one factor that will keep the abortion question before us in the future. Underlying all these differences can be identified a multidimensional ethical dilemma.

MEDICAL PROFESSION CONTEXT

The medical profession shared the anti-abortion mood prevalent in the United States during the latter part of the nineteenth century and may have influenced the enactment of stringent criminal abortion legislation. In 1857 the American Medical Association (AMA) appointed a Committee on Criminal Abortion to investigate criminal abortion with a view to its general suppression. In 1859 this committee proposed, and the AMA adopted, a resolution against unwarrantable destruction of human life. They called upon state legislatures to revise their abortion laws, and requested the cooperation of state medical societies in pressing the subject. The committee in 1871 again proposed resolutions that the AMA adopted. This time one recommendation read that it "be unlawful and unprofessional for any physician to induce abortion or premature labor without the concurrent opinion of at least one respectable consulting physician, and then always with a view to the safety of the child—if that be possible." They also recommended calling "the attention of the clergy of all denominations to the perverted views of morality entertained by a large class of females—aye, and men also, on this important question."[40]

Except for occasional condemnation of criminal abortionists, the AMA took no further formal action on abortion until 1967, when the Committee on Human Reproduction urged adoption of a policy in which the Association would oppose induced abortion except where (1) documented medical evidence showed a threat to the health or life of the mother, (2) the child may be born with incapacitating physical deformity or mental deficiency, or (3) a pregnancy resulting from legally established statutory or forcible rape or incest may constitute a threat to the physical or mental health of the patient. In addition, the committee proposed that two other physicians with recognized professional competency examine the patient and concur in writing as to the need for the abortion and that the physician perform the abortion in a hospital accredited by the Joint Commission on Accreditation of Hospitals. The AMA House of Delegates adopted this policy.[41] In 1970, the resolutions before the House of Delegates did not differ from the policy adopted in 1967 with the exception of the statement that "no party to the procedure should be requested to violate personally held moral principles."[42]

THE SCIENTIFIC CONTEXT

Science, like religion, finds it difficult to establish the moment when life begins. One embryologist could define the unfertilized egg as a living entity but another embryologist could indicate great limitations in that definition because the unfertilized egg cannot continue to live more than a few days, has only half the chromosome supply that other body cells have and therefore it cannot develop without the addition of the sperm. This situation changes the moment an egg becomes impregnated by a male sperm and this change results in a complete chromosome supply. The process of division begins and growth occurs rapidly; however, up to the sixth week of its existence, only an expert embryologist can tell whether this embryo is human or not. At the seventh week, human characteristics begin appearing and by the 15th or 16th week the mother can feel the movements of the fetus.

All along the way of this remarkable process the embryo has what some call the marvelous gift of life but others would argue that this is true only in the same sense that an animal or plant has life. The question remains as to when during this process this entity develops human life. No clear and biological definition has been developed as to the beginning of human life.

THE SOCIAL CONTEXT

In the years preceding the Supreme Court decision, dissatisfaction developed among physicians, legislators, judges, lawyers, and others regarding what they define as the archaic abortion laws. Specifically, these dissatisfactions focused on (1) a decision for abortion based on and limited to maternal survival, while health and well-being receive no consideration; (2) the complete failure to grant importance to the quality of the offspring, (3) no heed given to the circumstances under which impregnation occurs; and (4) the system under which abortion can be obtained invites inequities among those aborted.[43]

On one end of the abortion controversy, the group that wants more reform proposes that abortion should be a decision of the woman alone, or in consultation with her physician and that the procedure should be performed in any public or private facility with no legal statute imposing penalties on any party involved. This position assumes that no woman should bear any child she does not want, regardless of her reason and that no legal statute or medical committee should interfere in her personal decision. The proponents of this position have used it to demonstrate how conservative the new abortion law is when judged by this group's position. In developing the argument for the woman's right to her personal decision about abortion, the only criterion would be consistent with the individual woman's personal set of moral and religious values and in the final analysis only she can judge that.

Rossi believes that buried deeply beneath the abortion discussion one finds unresolved attitudes toward sex in this country. In addition, and perhaps compounding this situation, Americans seem to have a high tolerance for discrepancies between the moral norms they profess adherence to and what they privately practice and believe.[44] The National Opinion Research Center in 1965 conducted a survey asking a representative sample of 1484 adults in this country their views on the conditions under which a woman should be able to obtain a legal abortion. The major findings revealed widespread support among a majority of adults for legal abortion when a pregnancy involved a risk to maternal health, sexual assault, or probability of deformity in the fetus. The analysis of these data in terms of religious groups and sex difference showed that the important variable was not religion or sex per se, but the association of the two variables with church attendance. In other words, the more closely women and men, Catholic and Protestant, were involved with religion, the greater their tendency to reject a liberal stand on abortion.[45]

The groups that believe that abortion can be morally justified do not wish to force women or health professionals who define it as morally wrong to participate in the procedure against their will. However, they do not wish to be denied the abortion choice, with the result of forcing women into childbearing against their will.[46] If women have access to abortion, the moral choice can be made; if, however, society denies this access, then the moral choice becomes determined for all by the values of some.

On the other end of the abortion controversy, we have the group that would make abortion illegal and inaccessible, except perhaps under highly specified circumstances having to do with saving the mother's life. Two major concerns have been voiced by this group regarding the effects of liberalizing the abortion laws. The first concern has to do with the effect undergoing an abortion will have on the individual woman and the second with the effects these laws will have on societal attitudes and behavior. As to the first concern, this group assumes that the more the abortion laws, the more women will seek and, in fact, undergo abortion. This action denies the fetus the right to life. They argue that while giving the woman self-determination, easily accessible legal abortion does not afford the same right to the fetus who cannot act in his own defense. The belief underlying this position places more weight on the benefit to society in keeping the legal presumption against abortion and less weight on the benefits to the prospective mother in being able to make her own decisions. One major component of this underlying belief focuses on the idea that to destroy the fetus, a human being, would diminish our reverence for life, our instinct for protecting the helpless, our concern that all forms of human life receive protection.[47] This position has little sociopsychological data with which to defend its position and cross-cultural comparisons do not instruct us fully regarding our own situation. However, the anti-abortion position and the pro-abortion position reflect the inherent strains in an irreducibly pluralist society and serve to bring into sharper focus the ethical dilemmas involved.

THE ETHICAL DILEMMA OF ABORTION

Since the 1973 Supreme Court decision making legal abortion more readily available, some believed that further ethical debate would only be academic in the most pejorative sense of that word. Others, however, believed that moral distinctions can be made within the framework of the reformed law and these distinctions can assist the individual in developing or maintaining a moral position on abortion. The ethical dilemma involved can be limited to three of its dimensions for the purpose of discussion: (1) the rights of the fetus, (2) the rights and obligations of the mother, and (3) the rights and obligations of society. The two moral principles, consent and autonomy, are at the core of this ethical dilemma.

Rights of the Fetus

In presenting the *Roe* v. *Wade* case before the Supreme Court, the lawyer argued that the Constitution does not define "person" in so many words. Although the 14th Amendment contains three references to "person," there can be no assurance that they have any prenatal application. The lawyer concluded that under the law the unborn fetus is not a person. But one important dimension of this ethical dilemma asks for a definition of human life and some determination of when we can recognize its presence, so that we can then place a value on it and weigh it against other values. In the present state of biologic ignorance on the matter and philosophical pluralism, the premise that the fetus is a person can neither be proved or disproved to the satisfaction of all. Therefore, no one can assert superior moral sensitivity over opponents, and neither moral claim can rightfully eliminate the other from the political arena.[48]

Those concerned with what they consider a helpless minority, the unborn fetus, judge the direct, intentional taking of innocent human life as an un-acceptable means, however desirable the ends. Western religions, which teach an inclusive love of all people, foster a reverence for life and a respect for its sacredness that encourages an attitude of hesitancy toward the abortion act. The Protestant theologian Paul Ramsey finds support in genetic research for the position that we should impute full human dignity to the nonviable fetus. Although not all ethicists would accept his moral reasoning, Ramsey argues that genetics tells us that we were what we became in every cell and attribute. Genetic data therefore provide us with a scientific approximation to the religious belief of ensoulment from conception.[49]

If we grant that from conception a fetus possesses humanity, we must then accord it all human rights including the most basic one, the right to life. To kill that which possesses humanity is murder except in the cases of war, self-defense, and capital punishment. Dealing with this, Bok's moral reasoning raises the larger question of whether the life of the fetus should receive the same protection as other lives. Basically, she asks the question: Is killing the fetus, by whatever means, and for whatever reasons, to be thought of as killing a human being? By drawing the line between abortions performed early in pregnancy and those done later, she develops the moral position that early abortions do not violate the principles of protection for life.[50]

One basic moral principle that has received much attention in recent years, that of informed consent, must be addressed in this dilemma. If one defines the fetus as possessing humanity at any point along the developmental continuum prior to birth, then the question must be asked: Who speaks for this human, using what criteria, and who guards his rights in this matter so vital to his existence? One argument, especially for the severely deformed fetus, says that if the fetus could speak for himself under these circum-stances, he would consent to abortion. This argument can also be used to support abortions for the unwanted child without deformity. If the parent(s) does not want the child, what quality of life can he expect to have? Will this child more likely become a victim of the increasing social problem, child abuse? The central question in the quality of life argument turns on the location of the line to be drawn. Will the line fall so as to include the variables of deformity, sex of fetus, color of hair and eyes as legitimate reasons for abortion?

Rights and Obligations of the Pregnant Woman

The other moral principle, autonomy, leads to the position that a woman has the right to her own body and the right to determine her own fertility. The dilemma arises out of the fact that the situation involves two lives. According to some, no one has an absolute, clear-cut right to control one's fate where others share it. The Court took this consideration into account in their debate prior to changing the abortion law and in making distinctions between what is allowed during the three trimesters as the embryo develops into a viable fetus.

Bok raises the question as to whether anyone, before or after birth, child or adult, has the right to continued dependence upon the bodily processes of another against the person's will.[51] Thompson cogently argues that a woman, pregnant as a result of rape or in spite of every precaution, has no obligation to continue the pregnancy. In this case the author equates abortion with cessation of continued support and not with unjust killing. An involuntarily pregnant woman can cease her support of life to the fetus without moral infringement of its right to life.[52] Even those who support this argument under the circumstances specified might have difficulty using it in the situation of pregnancies entered into voluntarily. In this latter situation the obligation of the pregnant woman to the fetus would be defined differently and abortion might be considered less of a viable moral choice.

The exception to the overriding obligation to the fetus argument in the case of voluntary pregnancies may be, at least for some, an abnormal fetus. Not only does this raise the issue of quality of life for the yet unborn child, but also for the parents and for other children, if any, in the family.

Thompson also draws attention to the fact that the major focus in writings on abortion has been on what a third party, such as a physician, may or may not do when a woman requests an abortion. What the pregnant woman may do legally and morally became deduced from what third parties may do in the situation. To treat the matter of what the pregnant woman may do in such a fashion does not grant to her the status of person that others insist on so firmly for the fetus. This comment finds grounding in the basic tenet of a democratic society that people must be permitted to exercise a maximum degree of individual freedom, bound only by a proper regard for the legitimate rights of other citizens.[53]

Little attention has been given to the role, rights, and obligations of the father in the abortion decision. That reflects the law's concern with the individual, in this case the pregnant woman.

Rights and Obligations of Society

One of the factors for any society in balancing values is the question of where to draw the line. In this case, that means under what conditions and considering the importance of the variables, will society determine its abortion policy. If society develops a fairly restrictive policy, then the argument could be made that some women would be threatened by the continuation of pregnancy, the new child would place great economic and psychologic burdens on the family, the mode of existence and the career of some women would be seriously disrupted, and physically or mentally damaged infants would be born.[54] On the other hand, if the policy permits women to obtain abortion with no restrictions or at least very limited restrictions, then the "wedge" argument can be brought into the discussion. This argument says that there may be good reasons adduced for doing or not doing something because of what may possibly or predictably follow. This then raises the following questions. What will come to be the case if our society does X? Will this social practice have consequences on other practices?[55] Applied to the abortion situation, the questions become as follows. If social policy makes abortion available, will this lead that society to diminish its reverence for life and possibly to a lessening of our collective instinct for protecting the helpless? Would one such policy lead to other policies affecting the elderly, the mentally ill, and the mentally retarded? Could such policies push a society into disregarding the life of others who may not be productive or who may be a burden on society, such as the chronically ill or the chronically unemployed? No data from other countries with liberal abortion practices such as Sweden and Japan support this argument.

On a planet as interrelated as our own, some have taken the position that population control has become an overriding problem affecting every society and have suggested abortion as one method to deal with this problem. Using demographic, economic, sociologic, and psychologic data, population experts have argued for and against abortion as an important means of birth control. One such expert has argued the issue from a moral perspective and on that basis has decided against abortion as a viable means of population control.[56]

The crux of the matter regarding abortion and the rights and obligations of society can be summarized by raising two questions. First, does society derive some benefits in legally and socially restricting abortion that override the benefits to the prospective mother of being able to make her own decisions? This question points out the need to balance the rights and obligations of society as a whole against the rights and obligations of the individual member of that society. Second, will the effects of our abortion policy be determined by the meaning that society attaches to abortion vis-à-vis its

definition of human life per se and its definition of the quality of life derived? One of the major stresses surrounding abortion remains the fact that
if abortions are not available then those who define this procedure as right
and good based on their value system are denied access to abortion because
of the value system of others who view it as wrong and bad. Some argue
that, with the availability of abortions, no one forces another to undergo
one against her own moral stand. The moral positions in any pluralistic
society tend to reflect many diverse values which can lead to intolerance
of other viewpoints. The question of how we live with each other and each
other's different values raises a central ethical dilemma.

ABORTION AND NURSING

A brief review of the nursing and related literature provided insight into
the activities and concerns of nurses as they have, in recent years, dealt with
the ethical dilemmas of abortion. In 1967 the *American Journal of Nursing*
(AJN) published a paper on abortion pointing out that as society's views
change, the law changes.[57] This reflected the ferment going on in the years
just prior to the Supreme Court decision. At the American Nurses' Association 1968 convention, the Division of Maternal and Child Health Nursing
Practice presented a Statement to Study State Abortion Legislation. The
delegates approved this statement with some discussion on whether the
organization should take a stand on such a controversial issue that might be
misunderstood. They expressed concern over the loose application of abortion laws that could result in serious risks to women and their families and
expressed support of movements to examine and modify existing abortion
laws.[58] At about the same time, an essay on nurses' attitudes and abortion
addressed the issue of personal moral positions and professional obligations.[59] During the late 1960s and early 1970s the AJN kept its readers
abreast of the changes occurring in the state abortion laws in this country and
of the changes and nurses' reactions to them in the United Kingdom. In
addition, it reported the proceedings of an interdisciplinary panel on abortion.[60] Throughout the early 1970s, the AJN reported activities and experiences of individuals and groups concerned with abortion.[61,62,63-65]
Occasionally, a paper presenting some aspect of nursing care and abortion
appeared.[66,67] In January 1972, the Journal editor, Thelma Schorr, said in
an editorial on abortion that "the search for moral values is part of what
makes one human. Respecting the rights of others in their search also makes
one humane."[68]

The research on nursing and abortion has focused, in the main, on attitudes.
One study reported that in a sample of 500 nurses, 23 percent favored

unrestricted abortion. Half or more favored abortion in cases of rape, defective fetus, physical or mental impairment of the woman, and grave economic hardship. Of the total, 75 percent stated that they would treat the abortion patient with as much understanding as any other patient.[69] Another study found older nurses and those at community hospitals less likely to condone abortion than their younger, university hospital counterparts.[70] A survey found that the kind and quality of involvement each health worker had had in dilemmas of unwanted pregnancy were important determinants of attitudes toward abortion. The organization and administration of abortion services and the social environment, including the attitude toward abortion in the general community and among professional peers, also affected the attitudes of health workers.[71] One year prior to the Court decision, research involving 50 nurses indicated that 22 did not favor a change in the law based on religious, ethical-professional, and social reasons.[72] A report sampling doctors and nurses who had actually participated in large numbers of abortions said that the doctor's involvement beyond the clinic and the operating room could be described as perfunctory. The nurses suffered considerable stress attempting to resolve their ambivalence about their participation in these procedures and reported some feelings of anxiety, depression, and anger toward patients for their sexual acting out.[73] When researchers compared the attitudes of social workers and nurses, they found that social workers evidenced more favorable attitudes toward abortion and explained the difference by the social structure of the two professions.[74] And finally, another study reported that significantly more nursing students and their faculty opposed abortion on demand than did other health professionals and the general population with comparable education. Fewer nursing students and faculty voiced willingness to help a client obtain an abortion than did other health professionals.[75]

From the research cited, it seems apparent that the individual nurse, and especially one who works in a setting where she will have contact with abortion patients, must come to know and to understand her own moral position on abortion. She may arrive at this position through religious belief or through her own ethical reasoning. Additionally, certain aspects of values have a fluidity and can change with new input and insight, so it becomes necessary for individuals to reassess their moral position.

If the nurse finds that because of her values she cannot condone abortion on any grounds, then the likelihood of her being able to care for an abortion patient without exhibiting unkind or even punitive behavior seems greatly diminished. In New York State, laws have been enacted that protect the individual who refuses to perform or participate in an abortion because this procedure is contrary to his/her conscience or religious beliefs. Such laws make the violation of this provision by an employer a misdemeanor. Furthermore, these laws indicate that no civil action for negligence or malpractice shall be maintained against a person refusing to perform or participate in an abortion. Every nurse confronted with this situation has both the right and the obligation to obtain information regarding state laws and institution policies on this matter.

A slightly more complicated situation may arise when a nurse approves of abortion for certain reasons but not for others, or when she believes abortion should be limited to the first trimester. Some nurses can work with patients admitted for a D-and-C procedure since these abortions occur early in their pregnancy, while these same nurses find it difficult, if not impossible, to work with patients aborted by the saline method since the fetus will be further along in development. If the type of patients admitted match the nurses' category of permissible abortion, then she should have no real ethical problems in providing nursing care; however, if they do not, she will need to work out a solution to her ethical dilemma in which her personal value system and her professional obligations conflict. A head nurse or nursing supervisor can play an important role here by discussing the issues with the staff nurse, provided her awareness of the ethical dilemma included the balancing of the rights of the nurse-as-person with the obligations of the nurse-as-professional.

Perhaps the most worrisome type of situation arises with the nurse who either has given little thought to her moral position on abortion or who denies to herself that she harbors resentment toward abortion patients in order to maintain her job. One can only hope that each nurse will seriously think about her beliefs as to the sanctity of life and where she can morally draw the line between what she thinks is right or wrong, have some understanding of how she reached her conclusion, and realize how this will affect what functions she can and can not perform based on this moral position.

In the last analysis, the nurse must arrive at a balance between her own values and her professional obligations to the patient. In the process of reasoning through the ethical dilemmas involved in abortion, the least that can be hoped is that she not add to the bureaucratic banality of suffering.[76] The most that can be hoped is that each nurse regard the rights of others as precious as she would want her own regarded and that within this context she view her obligations to herself, to the patient, to nursing, and to her place of employment.

REFERENCES

1. Kleinman RL: Abortion Classification and Techniques. London, International Planned Parenthood Federation, 1971, p 7
2. Hellman L, Pritchard J: Williams Obstetrics. New York, Appleton, 1971, p 493

3. Potts DM: Postconception control of fertility. Int J Gynecol & Obstet, November 1970, pp 957–70
4. Cook RE, Hellegers AE, Hoyt RG, Richardson HW (eds): The Terrible Choice: The Abortion Dilemma. New York, Bantam, 1968, pp 40–41
5. Guttmacher AF: Abortion—yesterday, today, and tomorrow. In Guttmacher AF (ed): The Case for Legalized Abortion Now. Berkeley, Calif, Diablo, 1967, pp 8–9
6. Tietze C, Lehfeldt H: Legal Abortion in Eastern Europe. JAMA 175: 1149–54, 1961
7. Tietze C, Abortion on request: its consequences for population trends and public health. In Stoane RB (ed): Abortion—Changing Views and Practice. New York, Grune & Stratton, 1971, pp 165–66
8. Gebhard PH, Pomeroy WB, Martin CE, Christenson CV: Pregnancy, Birth and Abortion. New York, Harper, 1958
9. Rainwater L: Family Design: Marital Sexuality, Family Size, and Contraception. Chicago, Aldine, 1965
10. Cartwright A: Parents and Family Planning Service. New York, Atherton, 1970
11. Westoff LA, Westoff CF: From Now to Zero. Boston, Little, Brown, 1971
12. Staples R: The sexuality of black women. Sexual Behavior 2:4–15, 1972
13. Russell KP, Jackson EW: Therapeutic Abortions in California. Am J Obstet Gynecol 105:757–65, 1969
14. Overstreet EW: California's abortion law—a second look. In Reiterman C (ed): Abortion and the Unwanted Child. New York, Springer, 1971, pp 15–26
15. Smith KD, Steinhoff PG, Diamond M, Brown N: Abortion in Hawaii: the first 124 days. Am J Public Health 61:530–42, 1971
16. Pakter J, Nelson F: Abortion in New York City: the first nine months. Fam Plann Perspect 3:5–12, 1971
17. Stone AA: The psychiatric dilemma. Human Sexuality 4:29, 32, February 1970
18. Pasnau RO: Medical Tribune, August 4, 1971
19. Blake J: Abortion and public opinion: the 1960–1970 decade. Science 171:540–49, 1971
20. Lipson G, Wolman D: Polling Americans on birth control and population. Fam Plann Perspect 4:39–42, January 1972
21. Saltman J, Zimering S: Abortion Today. Springfield, Ill, Thomas, 1973, p 101
22. Bok S: Ethics and decision making in medicine. Lecture at Harvard University, January 17, 1977
23. Powledge TM, Sollitto S: Prenatal diagnosis—the past and the future. Hastings Cent Rep, November 1974, pp 11–13
24. Lappé M: How much do we want to know about the unborn? Hastings Cent Rep, February 1973, pp 8–9
25. US Law Week 41:4213–4233, 1973 (*Roe* v. *Wade*)

26. Ibid: pp 4233–4240 (*Doe* v. *Bolton*)
27. Castiglioni A: A History of Medicine. New York, Aronson, 1973
28. Edelstein L: The Hippocratic Oath: Text, Translation, and Interpretation. Baltimore, Johns Hopkins University Press, 1967
29. Noonan JT: An almost absolute value in history. In Noonan JT (ed): The Morality of Abortion. Cambridge, Harvard University, 1970, p 4
30. Ibid: p 7
31. Gustafson JM: A Protestant ethical approach. In Noonan: JT: op cit, p 116
32. Ibid: p 119
33. Margolies IR: A Reform rabbi's view. In Hall RE (ed): Abortion in a Changing World. New York, Columbia University Press, 1970, vol 1. pp 30-33
34. Nazer IR: Abortion in the Near East. In Hall RE: op cit, p 268
35. Stern L: Abortion: reform and the law. J Crim Law 59:84, 1968
36. Louisell DW, Noonan JT: Constitutional balance. In Noonan JT: op cit, p 223
37. Saltman J, Zimering S: op cit, p 73
38. Heller A, Whittington HG: The Colorado story: Denver General Hospital experience with the change in the law on therapeutic abortion. Am J Psychiatr 125:809-16, 1968
39. Cook RE et al: op cit, pp 60-61
40. AMA: 22 Transcript. 258:1871
41. AMA: Proceedings of the House of Delegates. June 1967, pp 40-51
42. AMA: Proceedings of the House of Delegates. June 1970, p 221
43. Guttmacher AF: op cit, p 12
44. Rossi AS: Public views on abortion. In Guttmacher AF: op cit, pp 31-33
45. Ibid: pp 35-51
46. Pohlman E: Abortion dogmas needing research scrutiny. In Sloane RB: op cit, p 17
47. Cook RE et al: op cit, pp 65-66
48. Cook RE et al: op cit, p 82
49. Ramsey P: Points in deciding about abortion. In Noonan JT: op cit, p 67
50. Bok S: Ethical problems of abortion. Hastings Cent Rep January 1974, pp 33-52
51. Ibid, p 34
52. Thomson J: A defense of abortion. Philosophy and Public Policy 1:47-66, 1971
53. Group for the Advancement of Psychiatry: The Right to Abortion. New York, Scribner's, 1970, p 26
54. Brody B: Abortion and the Sanctity of Life. Cambridge, MIT Press, 1975, p 120
55. Noonan JT: op cit, pp 85-86
56. Dyck AJ: Is abortion necessary to solve population problems? In Hilgers

TW, Horan DJ (eds): Abortion and Social Justice. New York, Sheed and Ward, 1972, pp 159–76

57. Hershey N: As society's views change, laws change. Am J Nurs, November 1967, pp 2310–12
58. ANA convention: a week of "firsts." Am J Nurs, June 1968, p 1261
59. Fonseca JD: Induced abortion: nursing attitudes and actions. Am J Nurs, May 1968, pp 1022–27
60. Abortion. Am J Nurs, September 1970, pp 1919–25
61. Catholic nurse–legislator files for abortion reform. Am J Nurs, March 1971, p 459
62. Personal experience at a legal abortion center. Am J Nurs, January 1972, pp 110–12
63. Nurses' feelings a problem under new abortion law. Am J Nurs, February 1971, p 350
64. Nurses' Association of American College of Obstetricians and Gynecologists: principles and guidelines on abortion. Am J Nurs, July 1972, p 1311
65. Abortion yes or no; nurses organize both ways. Am J Nurs, March 1972, pp 416–18
66. Cronenwett LR, Choyce JM: Saline abortion. Am J Nurs, September 1971, pp 1754–57
67. Ketter C, Copeland P: Counseling the abortion patient is more than talk. Am J Nurs, January 1972, pp 102–6
68. Schorr TM: Issues of conscience. Am J Nurs, January 1972, p 61
69. What nurses think about abortion. RN, June 1970, pp 40–43
70. Brown NK, Thompson DJ, Bulger RJ, Laws EH: How do nurses feel about euthanasia and abortion? Am J Nurs, July 1971, pp 1413–16
71. Survey finds determinants of attitudes toward abortion. Am J Nurs, October 1971, p 1900
72. Branson H: Nurses talk about abortion. Am J Nurs, January 1972, pp 106–9
73. Kane FJ, Feldman M, Jain S, Lipton MA: Emotional reactions in abortion service personnel. Ach Gen Psychiatr, March 1973, pp 409–11
74. Hendershot GE, Grimm JW: Abortion attitudes among nurses and social workers. Am J Public Health, May 1974, pp 438–41
75. Rosen RAH, Werley HH, Ager JW, Shea FP: Some organizational correlates to nursing students' attitudes toward abortion. Nurs Res, May–June 1974, pp 253–59
76. Denes M: In Necessary and Sorrow: Life and Death in an Abortion Hospital. New York, Basic Books, 1976, p 14

7

DYING AND DEATH

INTRODUCTION

To talk about the dying and death of one individual is to talk about the life of everyone. Death is a common denominator for all living beings, try as we may to ignore or deny it. As a topic of research and discussion, death has received much attention in lay and professional literature.[1-6]

Nurses are involved with patients at all locations on the continuum from birth to death and with families and communities before the birth and after the death of individuals. Before the days of sophisticated life-support mechanisms and antibiotics, death was an event that might be questioned but was accepted as an inevitability. This is no longer the situation in today's society. The process of dying is often prolonged in hospitals, nursing homes, and other institutions where eight out of ten Americans die.[7]

Urgent questions arise as to when death actually occurs, the "quality of life" for an individual, active versus passive euthanasia as morally acceptable actions, and the individual's "right to die with dignity." Should the interests of the individual or of society prevail in deciding these issues? These questions confront health professionals with ethical dilemmas that have far-reaching implications for individuals, families, and the human community.

How should rights of the individual patient, the family, health workers, and the community be weighed in making a decision about a congenitally deformed infant who will die without a sequence of surgical interventions and the use of costly medical resources? Who should decide? Does an individual have the right to choose his own death? Can we distinguish meaningfully between ordinary and extraordinary means in maintaining and preserving life? For whom? Is there a moral difference between letting a person die and taking an action to hasten death?

The Karen Quinlan case and decision in New Jersey (1976) refocused some of these questions for health professionals, for other professions such as law and theology, and for the entire human community when it made the headlines in the various news media. Another situation that served a similar purpose was the death of a newborn with Downs' Syndrome and duodenal atresia at Johns Hopkins Hospital a few years earlier. The parents refused surgery and the infant was allowed to die by starvation. Subsequently, a film was made that has elicited hours of agonizing discussion and questioning by health professionals, students, and others who have viewed the film.[8]

Before considering various concepts of death, a continuum of modes of intervention in dying and death is presented in Table 2. These modes range from dying and death with no intervention from self or others (for example, an elderly person dying alone in a housing project apartment) to intervention by another who causes death by giving a lethal dose of a drug intravenously. The ethical, legal, medical, social, psychologic, and economic factors to be considered in types of intervention will vary with the individual and family involved, whether the person is a newborn child, adult, or elderly person;

Table 2. CONTINUUM OF INTERVENTION: DYING AND DEATH

Outside Institutional Setting: Dying and Death	Institutional Setting Prolonged Dying–Hastening Death		
No intervention from self or others	Intervention: use of ordinary and/or extraordinary measures by health professionals	Intervention: self, family members, or others; e.g., "right to die" and living will	Intervention: self (suicide)* or others (active or passive euthanasia)

*May also be outside institutional setting.

whether the person has access to a small, rural community hospital or a large teaching/research-oriented medical center. Decisions about types of intervention are extremely complex for everyone involved because of the numbers and kinds of factors intersecting in each individual situation. There are significant implications from the decisions made in individual situations for the community in terms of the moral principles of the characteristics of justice, fairness, equality, truth telling, beneficence, and wrong-making in the act of killing.

Thinking about decisions of intervention requires consideration of how and when biologic and social death is defined and determined for such actions as "pulling the plug" and taking organs from donors for those still living.

DEFINING AND DETERMINING DEATH

Death, according to *Webster's Third New International Dictionary* (1971) is the ending of all vital functions without possibility of recovery, the end of life, the act, process, or fact of dying, the state of being no longer alive, a tasteless, joyless, dull existence, and the state of being without full possession of enjoyment of the intellectual or physical faculties. Certainly one questions when an individual is actually *dead* with this tremendous range of definitions. This range, however, does imply the social, psychologic and physical dimensions of death. But which is determinant of death in the sense that one can say, X is dead? There is similar confusion with use of the word "dead." The definition ranges the continuum from having ended existence as a living or growing thing, being without power to move, feel, or respond, to incapable of feeling or being stirred emotionally or intellectually. Can one then be dead socially but not physically? This is a metaphysical question beyond the scope of this chapter. Both a process and an event are implied in these varied definitions. Tolstoy's novel, *The Death of Ivan Ilyich,* offers a telling description of the social, psychological, and physical aspects of death as a process for the individual and family. Again, these definitions raise all the questions mentioned previously and increase the complexity for those who make decisions about whether or not a machine should be unplugged or extraordinary measures begun for a particular individual.

Traditionally, it has been the physician who makes decisions concerning the dying patient. Fifty years ago, these decisions primarily involved the provision of comfort and reassurance for the patient and family. Today, Morison talks about three possible areas of decision making for the physician. With the trend toward "death with dignity," the patient is also involved in the choices of how to live while dying, the use of drugs to relieve pain, and the decision not to use medical measures that do not promote a cure. The three areas of decision making discussed by Morison are:

1. Using all possible means including "extraordinary" measures to keep the patient alive
2. Discontinuing "extraordinary" measures but continuing "ordinary" means
3. Taking some "positive" steps to hasten the individual's death or "speed its downward trajectory."[9]

In making these decisions, one must take into account such factors as the determination of what is "extraordinary" or "ordinary" in the means to be used for a given patient, for example, experimental drugs, complicated life-maintaining machines, antibiotics, and the need for organs by those awaiting transplants. This also raises the moral question of what factors should go into the equation by which a decision is made in any of the three areas. Patients may be perceived as being more valuable to the living if they can be declared dead in order that parts of their body, commonly corneas and kidneys, can be used for someone else. In this view, the patient is seen primarily as a means. In addition to factors already mentioned that may or may not enter into a decision of this nature, the "right to die" must also be taken into account. If one has the "right to life" at one end of the age spectrum, does not one also have the "right to die" at the other end?

While the dictionary definitions of death give us clues about the process of death, they do not help in determining "the moment" of death. The most prominent effort to update the definition of death is that of the Ad Hoc Committee of the Harvard Medical School reported in 1968.[10] This committee presented a definition of irreversible coma or brain death as a new criteria for biologic death in order to deal with some of the factors in the decision-making equation discussed above, e.g., "pulling the plug." This has since become known as the "Harvard criteria" or the "Harvard definition" of death. The committee came up with several determinations that are to be made only by a physician. A summary of these conditions follows:

1. Unreceptivity and responsivity, i.e., intensely painful stimuli evoke no response
2. No movements or breathing, i.e., observations are to be made for a period of at least one hour and if the patient is on a respirator, the respirator may be turned off for three minutes to determine whether there is any effort at spontaneous breathing
3. No reflexes
4. Flat electroencephalogram (EEG) recorded for a minimum of ten minutes and repeated at least 24 hours later with no change.

The validity of these determinations depends on no accompanying hypothermia or evidence of drug intoxication. The physician is to inform the patient's family, his/her colleagues, and nurses who have been involved with care of the patient when the determination of brain death has been made.[11] The committee emphasized that the patient should be declared dead before the respirator is turned off in order to provide physicians with a greater degree of legal protection.[12]

The state of Kansas legislated a definition of death based on ordinary standards of medical practice, including spontaneous brain function.[13] An editorial in the *New York Times* (March 2, 1977) stated that twelve states have passed laws that define death in terms of brain death. The Harvard definition and the Kansas statute provide guidelines, one legal, and a process for determining that biologic death has occurred. Judge Muir's decision in the Karen Quinlan case declared that physicians' decisions are controlling in the care of dying patients.[14] The decision remains primarily with medicine even though the Supreme Court of New Jersey modified the Muir decision to physicians making decisions about discontinuing use of life support mechanisms in consultation with an ethics committee.[15]

Questions about the precision and effectiveness of the brain death definitions are raised by various authors.[16-18] Even though these updated definitions exist, ethical questions can still be raised about a medical technology that depends on organ donors for transplants. If an individual is kept "alive" through artificial means, i.e., the heart beats and the blood circulates, but the patient's organs deteriorate. When death is finally pronounced, the organs may no longer be suitable for transplant. What are the rights of the individuals waiting for transplants?

Morison raises questions about attempting to determine a specific time of death when "life" in any organism, including man, is not a clearly defined entity with sharp beginning and end points.[19] This view of life is particularly clear in the abortion issue and the beginning of life. Could it be that different at the end of life? Morison sees human organisms as a complex interaction among individual cells, the totality of cells, and the environment.[20] The human system does not usually fail as a unit and so we may have to make judgments about the value and intactness of the complex interactions of the organism. Life is a continuous rather than a discontinuous process. According to Callahan, the issue cannot be settled by appeals to absolute rights or standards.[21] To some extent the process of dying today is partially controlled by individual human beings by use of available technologies. With this relative control comes the necessity to think very carefully about who should be involved in decisions relating to this control and again what goes into the equation used for decision making.[22]

Kass does not think that Morison offers sufficient evidence for his view on the continuity of life and says that the organism does die as a whole.[23]

Therefore, there is still validity for the concept of death as an event and for using "reasonable criteria" for determining that a person has died.[24] These two viewpoints, presented very briefly, again give the reader some notion of the complex philosophical, biologic, and social issues involved in decisions made about death and the dying process in a sophisticated medical technology. A patient-centered ethic requires that the individual patient remain the center of decision making until a social consensus is reached, if possible, on the factors that should be considered and weighed in the best interests of both the individual and the human community. All of these issues and questions seem to turn around the question of euthanasia and whether life does cease to be worth living in the sense that it is dying that is being prolonged, rather than the maintenance of meaningful living. A related question becomes: Should we use technology because it is available? Does man use technology as a means to human ends or is technology an end in and of itself?

EUTHANASIA AS AN ETHICAL DILEMMA: SOME LEGAL DIMENSIONS

The concept of euthanasia comes from the Greek meaning good or pleasant death. Is death ever preferable to life for an individual? For society? Is there any greater difference in "letting die" or killing, particularly in light of the moral law that thou shalt not kill? At the present time, there is no agreement on the answer(s) to these questions. One needs to look carefully at what the best interests are for a given patient in a specific situation and to distinguish this from the interests of the hospital and of society. The following discussion focuses primarily on the dying adult patient and on ethical, as distinct from religious, considerations per se. In attempting to provide at least tentative solutions to the initial question, Bok suggests an examination of the criteria for decision making as a first step:

1. Who decides? The physician, guardian, patient, family member, clergyman, and/or a committee?
2. For whom does one decide? self, proxy, or other?
3. What criteria are used?
4. With what degree of consent by the "victim"?[25]

One may also consider the moral principles involved, for example, justice, beneficence, and truth telling. Are they being violated by particular alternative decisions proposed? In considering question 4, Bok states that euthanasia should be considered only in relation to those who can ask to die. This eliminates newborns and infants, who represent a different moral situation.[26] It also becomes more problematic for those individuals "kept alive" on machines who are *non compos mentis,* i.e., not of sound mind.

Physicians Duff, Campbell, and Shaw, and Richard McCormick, a theologian, take another position in relation to newborns and argue that certain severely deformed newborns should be allowed to die by withdrawing or withholding treatment. These authors feel that these decisions should be made by the parents and their professional advisors, usually physicians, since they are most familiar with the complexities of a given situation.[27-29] These writers represent yet another point of view on decision making when euthanasia is considered. The reader already knows of other views mentioned in the earlier section on defining and determining death. These views suggest the confusion and conflict in attempting to answer the questions posed for the decision maker.

In looking at questions related to euthanasia, one sees a continuum of intervention for decision makers ranging from a strict "sanctity of life" or anti-euthanasia view through passive (inactive) euthanasia to active euthanasia. The anti-euthanasia position commits one to vigorous treatment with ordinary means. Extraordinary or heroic measures may be withheld, not started. There is much difficulty in determining what constitutes ordinary and extraordinary means because physicians and hospitals have different standards. Situations vary with the individual.

One author has defined *ordinary* means of preserving life as all medicines, treatments, and surgical procedures that offer a reasonable hope of benefit to a patient and can be obtained and used without excessive pain, expense or other inconveniences. *Extraordinary* means are those that are very costly, unusual, difficult, or dangerous, or do not offer a reasonable hope of benefit to the patient at a given time and place.[30] Could these definitions be used equally in a large teaching hospital and a small community hospital, or does it depend on where the dying individual finds himself as a patient? What may be considered ordinary treatment for one patient may be considered extraordinary for another patient, for example, the use of antibiotics for a patient with pneumonia and their use for the patient who has terminal cancer with metastasis to the brain and liver who develops pneumonia.

In passive or inactive euthanasia, commonly known as "letting die," treatment may not be initiated, ongoing treatment may be stopped, with or without the consent of the patient.[31] These are measures, commonly used in hospitals, that are now openly recognized by the development of guidelines for orders not to resuscitate.[32] Active euthanasia includes such actions as giving the patient the means to kill himself and directly bringing about the patient's death with or without consent.[33]

Where do patient "rights" to control one's dying fit into this consideration of euthanasia? Does a person have the "right to die" in a hospital committed to preserving life? Can one refuse life-saving treatment? It has been said that inhumanity is the "enemy," not death per se.[34] One feels the definite lack of any clear-cut guidelines in this area, although there is increasingly more action by various groups advocating legislation for "death with dignity," that is, free from pain and in relative control of how one ends life.

According to Florida attorney Simons, there is no provision in the law that compels a competent person to seek medical care, except where the illness is a threat to the public, for example, a communicable disease. In the case of *Palm Springs General Hospital, Inc.* v. *Martinez,* the hospital and the attending physician were not required to perform surgery or transfusions against the patient's will.[35] There have been contradictory findings in various cases where individuals refused life-saving blood transfusions due to religious beliefs, for example, the case of *Kennedy Memorial Hospital* v. *Heston* [58 N.J. 576, 279 A. 2d 670 (1972)], in which it was said that hospital ethics required life-saving treatment. In *Erickson* v. *Dilgard* [252 N.Y.S. 2d 705 (1962)], on the other hand, it was found that the patient did have the right to refuse a blood transfusion even though the patient would most likely die without it. One's right to "choose death" is confused legally.

In the Karen Quinlan case, Judge Muir said that, when an adult is rendered incompetent, society expects that the attending physician's decision will prevail even when there is a conflict with a family decision.[36] Judge Muir's decision conflicts with that of a national public opinion poll. When asked about a patient dying in the hospital with no hope of cure, over 50 percent of the sample said that it was all right to let the person die, i.e., passive euthanasia, and that the decision should be made by family members or the physician with family members. Only 7 percent felt that it was the decision of the patient's physician alone.[37] Physicians seem to agree with the public rather than with Judge Muir. In 1973, the AMA House of Delegates adopted a statement that condemned physicians agreeing to perform mercy-killing, but said that the stopping of extraordinary means to prolong the life of the body is the decision of the patient and/or his immediate family with freely available advice and judgment of the physician.[38] Commonly, "mercy killing" has been used to refer to active euthanasia.* One senses that a general social consensus is developing that physicians should not be the only individuals to make decisions about initiation of actions for aiding an individual's death.

In using the term euthanasia some authors make a distinction between mercy killing as active euthanasia and allowing people to die as passive euthanasia. One is an act of commission; the other, an act of omission, a

*See other physician opinions in references 27 and 29.

distinction between voluntary and involuntary euthanasia. Others consider euthanasia as any act done by another that results in hastening death for a suffering individual. There is no moral distinction between active and passive euthanasia. Acts of omission are seen as not interfering with the natural process of dying, while euthanasia as mercy killing is seen as inducing death as in the AMA House of Delegates' statement. Another distinction is that the "right to die" is associated only with the individual, while euthanasia demands that someone else, or society, intervene to induce death. This raises the question as to whether society should accept such an obligation.[39]

In the United States there are some serious gaps in the law for dealing with the broad issue of euthanasia. Consent or request for euthanasia is not legally acceptable as a defense. However, the law does take into account whether the question involved is an act or an omission; thus the law makes the distinction between active and passive euthanasia to some extent. According to Fletcher, there is no case in the Anglo-American tradition of law in which a physician has been convicted of murder or manslaughter for having killed to end the suffering of a patient.[40] This tradition, then, seems to consider intent of the physician. Nevertheless, confusion still exists as to the legal outcome in any specific situation.

There are at least three different ethical points of view on euthanasia that are significant to the nurse, other health professionals, and society in articulating a moral position on both active and passive euthanasia. One position, sometimes called the "new morality," supports a value system that puts humanness and personal integrity above biologic life and functions. This position stems from the ancient Christian-European belief that the core of humanness lies in man's rational faculty, that is, his cerebral function. What counts ethically as right-making action is whether or not human needs come first. The moral defense is that euthanasia helps the patient die rather than prolonging a slow, ugly, dehumanized death. This position holds the value that death is not the worst that can happen to an individual. Both Eastern and Western religions agree that one is not morally obliged to preserve life in all terminal cases. The Pope said as long ago as 1957 that it was not necessary to use "extraordinary" means to prolong life of the terminally ill.[41]

One objection to the general idea of euthanasia is that the same thing will happen as happened in Nazi Germany, a kind of "wedge" argument. Kohl sees this particular "wedge" argument as claiming that if beneficent euthanasia, a kindly act, can be morally justified then euthanasia for other purposes may be practiced and justified.[42] This kind of thinking is ignorant of the fact that the Nazis engaged in genocide and killing for experimental purposes, not "mercy killing" in the sense of a merciful act of kindness.[43] On the other hand, one should not ignore the findings of research in which, for example, a sample of university students were asked a variety of questions related to euthanasia and a "final solution" to problems of overpopulation and misery. Over half of the respondents said that "unfit" persons should be killed by society as a "final solution."[44] Fletcher feels that it is still more difficult to morally justify letting someone die a slow dehumanized death than not letting him do so. For Fletcher the practice of euthanasia as merciful killing implies compassion on the part of the agent and society. Others do not agree because killing for them always has wrong-making characteristics, even in self-defense.

In considering whether or not the end justifies the means, Fletcher uses the principle of "proportionate good," the balance of benefits and harms of an action for the suffering individual. A reminder of the Rawlsian criteria for moral principles follows, to be used in deciding whether or not one can morally justify the "proportionate good" principle for any form of euthanasia. A moral principle should be (1) *general* in the sense that it expresses general properties and relationships and is not specific to individual persons or relationships; (2) *universal* in the sense that it applies to everyone and is chosen with a view of consequences if everyone complies; (3) *public* in the sense that everyone knows and recognizes the principle as operative in society; (4) an *imposition of order* on conflicting claims in terms of using justice and right to make the adjustment rather than the capacity to coerce; and (5) *final* in the sense that this is the last court of appeal and overrides law, custom, social rules, and self-interest.[45] One may question whether the "proportionate good" principle meets all these criteria. One can also question why these criteria should be used, an issue that goes far beyond the scope of this discussion. One could say that this principle is in line with a "quality of life" ethic, which says that some lives are not worth living and can be taken. One is still left with the Biblical injunction, Thou shalt not kill.

Dyck argues for an ethic of benemortasia, which comes from the Latin, meaning good or kind death. This is an ethic of obligation and is concerned with how we should behave toward those who are dying or whose death appears to be a merciful event. Mercy is considered as a moral obligation in this position. What is the most morally responsible way to act in the face of one's own or another's death? In the face of continuing heated debate by proponents of beneficent euthanasia and opponents against it, the ethic of benemortasia suggests the following kind of care for patients who are considered to be "imminently dying": (1) the relief of pain; (2) the relief of suffering; (3) respect for the right of an individual to refuse treatment; and (4) universal provision of health care in the sense that individuals and families would not have to bear alone the burden of catastrophic medical care.[46]

A third position on euthanasia as "mercy killing" states that mercy killing as active euthanasia is never permissible and that treatment of people with respect is the fundamental principle of medical ethics. This position does make a moral distinction between killing and allowing to die. Disease is accepted as a cause of death, but a human agent should not be the cause of death according to this position. This seems to actually rule out both active and passive euthanasia. Another difference is between not actively fighting death and actively putting an end to life. Again, a further argument is that the starting point for considering the morality of any kind of killing is that evil is always present in the act of killing.

This third position holds that the physical element cannot be separated and excluded from what makes a person a person. A person is not just cerebral function. How does one determine what is "a person" for decision-making purposes? Weber says that the "sanctity of life" ethic should not be put aside in favor of a "quality of life" ethic as it will weaken man's respect for man, a dehumanizing ethic dangerous to human community.[47] This fear and other objections are expressed by various authors in considering whether and what kind of legislation should be enacted in this area.[48-50] What is best for the individual? What is best for society, now and in the future? These interests conflict in the euthanasia issue.

Weber goes on to say in the third view that there does come a time to cease prolonging life and to concentrate on needs of the dying person in an attempt to provide a peaceful death for the overall good of the individual patient. However, he warns that the physician must also be aware that the medical good of the patient is not always what the patient wants.[51] What the patient wants may change over time, making decisions even more slippery and leaving one open to mistakes.[52] A further complication is that the physician may have developed an ethic, expressed through the practice of "defensive medicine," which makes the physician insist that it is his duty to preserve life as long as possible. Consequences to the patient are not considered, but the physician hopes to avoid any future criticism for stopping life support mechanisms too soon.[53] So there are patients who are dead by the brain death criteria, but still kept "alive" by technological means.

In discussing the decision not to resuscitate, Weber says that this decision is fully compatible with respect for the intrinsic value of human life. He views this decision as a refusal to attempt to control life and death any further through the use of technology.[54] Two hospitals in the Boston area have reported on their efforts to develop guidelines for making the decision not to resuscitate.[55,56]

Further efforts to clarify the position of individuals and society on the "right to die with dignity" are seen in the development of living wills by a variety of individuals and groups including the Euthanasia Educational Council.[57] The living will prepared by the Euthanasia Educational Council has been used as a model for "death with dignity" bills introduced into state legislatures. One example in an article by Sisella Bok is presented here in its entirety:[58]

DIRECTIONS FOR MY CARE

I, _____, want to participate in my own medical care as long as I am able. But I recognize that an accident or illness may someday make me unable to do so. Should this come to be the case, this document is intended to direct those who make choices on my behalf. I have prepared it while still legally competent and of sound mind. If these instructions create a conflict with the desires of my relatives, or with hospital policies or with the principles of those providing care, I ask that my instructions prevail, unless they are contrary to existing law or would expose medical personnel or the hospital to a substantial risk of legal liability.

I wish to live a full and long life, but not at all costs. If my death is near and cannot be avoided, and if I have lost the ability to interact with others and have no reasonable chance of regaining this ability, or if my suffering is intense and irreversible, I do not want to have my life prolonged. I would then ask not to be subjected to surgery or resuscitation. Nor would I then wish to have life support from mechancal ventilators, intensive care services, or other life prolonging procedures, including the administration of antibiotics and blood products. I would wish, rather, to have care which brings comfort and support, which facilitates my interaction with others to the extent that this is possible, and which brings peace.

In order to carry out these instructions and to interpret them, I authorize _____ to accept, plan, and refuse treatment on my behalf in cooperation with attending physicians and health personnel. This person knows how I value the experience of living, and how I would weigh incompetence, suffering, and dying. Should it be impossible to reach this person, I authorize _____ to make such choices for me. I have discussed my desires concerning terminal care with them, and I trust their judgment on my behalf.

In addition, I have discussed the following specific instructions regarding my care:

(please continue on back)

Date _____   Signed _____

Witnessed by _____ and by _____

Bok suggests that each individual try to write his own living will in order to gain some understanding of the complexities in doing this. One problem often raised in relation to living wills is that the person may feel differently when writing the will and later when ill. What decision should be considered?

The Natural Death Act (1976) in California recognizes the right of adults to prepare written instructions authorizing their physicians to withhold or withdraw life-sustaining procedures in specified circumstances of terminal illness. A major purpose of the original bill was to settle a number of legal issues arising from "living wills" concerned with professional liability and insurance coverage. This Act relieves physicians, health facilities, and other licensed health professionals from civil liabilities for carrying our directives as defined in the bill. The bill declares that death resulting from carrying out a directive does not constitute suicide thus resolving this issue in relation to insurance polices as well.[59] A "living will" is legally binding in the state of California under stated conditions, the first state to legislate in this complex area. Other states are considering legislation in this area. While this legislation provides answers and guidelines for some problems, it has always been recognized that public policy of this import will raise a host of additional issues in relation to interpretation, for example.

Another piece of legislation in the area of death and dying is the Uniform Anatomical Gift Act that has passed in most of the states. This Act authorizes the gift of all or a part of a human body to be used after death for certain specified purposes.[60]

Previous discussion of the problem of active euthanasia and passive euthanasia as "allowing to die" focused primarily on adult and elderly patients. These issues were mentioned only briefly in relation to severely deformed newborns and children with terminal illness. Many of the same issues and questions involving adults apply to children and newborns. The basic issue when children and infants are involved is, Who should make the decision? Physician? Parents? Child? One may again ask the question as to whether or not a society should even consider allowing children to die, whether active or passive euthanasia is involved. What are the implications for individuals and the human community again in terms of the value of life? Some see this as a question of infanticide, others as a "quality of life" issue.[61-65] Engelhardt sees other special questions arising in relation to euthanasia and young children, for example, legal standing of the rights of children, status of parental rights, and obligations of adults to prevent suffering in children.[66] All of these questions are hotly debated wherever severely deformed infants and terminally ill children receive care. What are ordinary and extraordinary measures in a newborn intensive care unit? Does it depend on the available technology? The same question re-emerges: Do health professionals have obligations to use the technology available without looking at how lives are affected by it now and in the foreseeable future?

In summary, this brief overview of some of the issues and complexities of decision making related to euthanasia, death, and dying does not provide us with any answers. What it does do is give the reader some idea of directions taken by individuals, institutions, and society in seeking ways to make better decisions for all of us in this area. Before leaving the discussion of euthanasia, a short section will consider some issues related to ethics and suicide, sometimes called voluntary euthanasia, i.e., intervention by the self in causing one's own death.

SUICIDE AS AN ETHICAL DILEMMA

Suicide, or voluntary euthanasia, has been seen as an affirmation of life, a denial of life, and a questioning of life. The traditional religious teachings of the West since St. Augustine have condemned all forms of self-destruction.[67] Suicide was and still is considered by some to be a sin and an interference with God's will.

According to Kant man does not have the power of disposal of his body. One can only treat his body as he chooses related to self-preservation.[68] These views are being challenged in today's society, as they always have been to some extent in all societies.[69] One example is the Act of 1961 that declared that suicide should no longer be a crime.[70] Suicide is the tenth leading cause of death in the United States, with approximately 25,000 deaths per year. Annual attempts at suicide may range as high as 400,000.[71]

Murphy, a psychiatrist, talking about the right to commit suicide says that "rational" suicide may be ascribed to those persons suffering from a terminal disease. However, the majority of persons who commit suicide are not in this group. The majority suffer from clinically recognizable psychiatric illnesses and have sought help from physicians. Only a few have received necessary treatment.[72] Some light is thrown on this by a study done in the early 1970s that found that 75 percent of all suicides have consulted a physician before their act. Another finding was that the physician respondents had inadequate knowledge of suicide, e.g., the majority did not know the most vulnerable age group and many had negative attitudes toward suicide and people who attempted it.[73]

Heifetz, a neurosurgeon, states that under certain circumstances the group who are severely ill, near death, and who wish to commit suicide should receive help from their physician. Laws exist in Uruguay, Switzerland, Peru, Japan, and Germany for such assistance by the physician.[74] Such laws do not exist in the United States. However, Heifetz points out that this group must be separated from the lonely, the elderly, or physically handicapped who may also seek to commit suicide and ask another's assistance.[75]

The question of the individual's right to self-determination is a basic consideration in talking about the ethical dimensions of suicide. There are positions on both ends of the continuum, from Szasz's position that the individual has the right to self-determination and that he should retain this right even if the individual is considered by some to be potentially dangerous or suicidal to the view that the physician has the obligation to support "the desire for life" that exists even in those who feel that this desire has left them, e.g., individuals suffering from depression.[76,77] Other major arguments against suicide are that it is a crime against society, cowardly, a violation of one's duty to God, unnatural, an insult to human dignity, and that it is cruel because it inflicts pain upon one's family and friends. Hook suggests that this last argument, while not absolute, has greater weight than any of the previous arguments.[78]

Sometimes suicide is ethically justifiable. There is no categorical imperative that says one is to live but to live well. From this one can say that no rational morality would require that certain lives be continued in the face of disastrous accidents of birth or illnesses for which there are no effective remedial measures. Another aspect is that no social morality can be equally binding on everyone in society unless there is more equality in distributing the necessities, sometimes called the goods, of life.[79] One thinks in terms of justice and fairness, and the equal distribution of society's benefits and harms. The obligation seems to rest with those who say that one should not commit suicide to provide a just society in which all can "live well."

In summary, the question of suicide is extremely controversial in our society and raises many ethical questions for the health professional about the individual's right to self-determination versus the right of the human community to preserve itself. Whose rights should prevail in the face of conflict? Could the individual who commits suicide be performing a moral act under certain conditions? What conditions?

IMPLICATIONS FOR NURSING PRACTICE

Eight out of ten Americans die in hospitals, nursing homes, or other institutions where nurses are employed.[80] The nursing literature focuses primarily on attitudes toward death and dying patients, the depersonalized, institutionalized dying process, and the nurse's personal experiences with dying patients and their families.[81-89] Little has been written on the ethical dilemmas faced by nurses in relation to the dying patient, the family, and other health professionals, particularly the physician. Nurses can and should examine their own individual values in relation to death, "quality of life," the importance of individual needs of patients, and the moral principles of justice, beneficence, autonomy, and self-determination for the dying patient, and the ethical difference, if any, between "letting a patient die" or actively doing something to hasten the death of a particular patient.

Hershey, a lawyer, says that the nurse's legal responsibility is to respect the medical decision.[90] But one issue that frequently arises for the nurse is that she does not have specific orders on which to relie. Decisions must be made for specific patients when guidance has not been provided and cannot be obtained when a specific crisis arises. This will undoubtedly leave the nurse wondering if her action was "right" or "best" for a given patient, for example, in a cardiac arrest situation. These issues become even more complex for the nurse practitioner who may have responsibility for decisions whether to provide a life-preserving service, thus increasing the legal risk for the individual.[91] What are the professional and moral obligations of the nurse practitioner in these situations? What are the obligations of nurses in nursing homes where they may be the only daily resource for patients and families?

One example of hospital efforts to recognize a patient's right to refuse available medical procedures, in light of the hospital's primary philosophy to preserve life, is the development of guidelines for orders not to resuscitate mentioned in a previous section of this chapter. According to these guidelines, physicians have the primary obligation to explore the implications of this decision with the patient and family, but the initial judgment should be discussed first with the other physicians, nurses, and any others directly involved with the patient's care.[92] This provides an opportunity for nursing to add its assessment of a patient to those of others in the decision-making process and to carry out the *caring* process for dying patients. It is again the responsibility of the physician not only to record the order not to resuscitate but to convey the meaning of this order for a particular patient to medical, nursing and other appropriate staff.[93] Nurses are most likely in a key position to notify the physician if the patient's condition changes so that the orders no longer seem applicable.

Nurses should also be involved in the emotional support needed by the patient's family as they are often the only daily resource for families. One wonders then if it is unethical for nurses not to include this as part of their professional obligations to the patient, whether an adult or child. Various authors discuss how nurses can be most helpful to families of dying patients.[94, 95] Research has identified some needs of spouses of dying patients.[96] These needs are to be with the dying patient, to be helpful to the dying person, to be assured of the comfort of the dying person, to be informed of the mate's condition, to be informed of impending death, to be able to ventilate emotions, to have the comfort and support of other family members, and to have the acceptance, support, and comfort from health professionals. Half of the study sample reported that they did not have this last need met. Spouses generally agreed that nurses had been helpful to their dying mates but were too busy to help families. Nurses can be facilitators for meeting most of these needs, even in intensive care settings, by making themselves available to families. This is not without strain and tension for the nurse.[97, 98] The next question is whether nursing administration has an obligation to provide support systems for nursing staff involved with critically ill and dying patients.

Another issue facing nurses in many hospitals is the patient who arrives on the unit with a "living will" attached to the chart in a state where these wills are not legally binding. What if this presents a conflict, as it often does, between the autonomy and authority of the patient and that of the physician? This is one example of an issue in which an interdisciplinary board or committee constituted at the institutional level to discuss ethical issues could be most helpful.[99] Nurses can and should be actively participating in these groups, as they are a primary resource to their patients and because they confront so many of these issues in their daily practice.

Smith suggests that groups, when discussing issues of care for the dying, often fall into two categories: those with the "participant" point of view and those with the "administrative" perspective.[100] Nurses and physicians are usually in the first group, that is, they often identify with the patient and what they assume to be in the best interests of the patient. The second perspective views the dying patient as a managerial problem and is more concerned, for example, with the use of hospital resources. Problems follow from these two viewpoints. The "participant" perspective in advocating death with dignity and rights of patients to refuse treatment often ignores when and under what circumstances patients should choose death. Health professionals must also guard against imposing their own values on patients and families. The "administrative" viewpoint is concerned with efficient use of resources and the equality of treatment for all patients, thus ignoring the diversity of individual patient needs.[101]

Ramsey warns that in disagreements between these viewpoints questions should be resolved as *patient* policy questions, not as hospital or public policy questions in terms of limited beds or other hospital resources, for example.[102] The danger exists that more and more decisions will be based on numbers and needs that can be accomodated or on a utilitarian ethic that considers the greatest happiness for the greatest number as the determinant in decision making. In light of this, one needs to refocus on the ethic that says "do no harm" and on Frankena's moral principles of justice (equal treatment) and beneficence for patients and families, with both common and individual needs considered.[103]

Authors Smith, Dyck, and Ramsey emphasize the importance of *caring* for the dying when the person is beyond the point where life can be preserved.

Smith sees nurses and other health professionals as "healers and menders" of patients. He makes the significant point, however, that in caring for patients there are some dimensions of the patient's life that are beyond the professional's appropriate concern. These concerns are more appropriate to the concern and attention of the family or the patient's "significant others" because they are most intimately involved with the patient.[104] This raises questions about decision making in caring for the individual who does not have others who form an immediate intimate unit of concern when those particular problems that concern only the patient and this unit arise and when it is inappropriate for health professionals to intervene.

Ramsey, discussing what he calls "premortem care," says that there is a duty, a categorical imperative, to never abandon *care*.[105] He says that in caring for the dying one may eventually cease doing what was once called for and begin to do what is now required in the individual situation. This does not mean, according to Ramsey, that one is required to assist the dying process, but to assure the person that they are not alone, that others are aware of their dying, and will be with them during the dying process. These caring values and practices are most clearly demonstrated in the hospice movement.[106] Ramsey also notes that we could formulate a moral rule that the *only* circumstances in which positive action might be taken to hasten a person's death is if there is the kind of prolonged dying where it is medically impossible to control the individual's pain, for example, in dying from bone cancer. The nurse, through close contact in caring for the patient, may be the first to assess that this situation has been reached by a particular patient. It becomes imperative for the nurse to communicate this to the patient's physician in an ethic of caring. The ethic and practice of allowing to die, recognized by most health professionals, still leaves us with the question as to whether physicians can take positive action to hasten death without weakening medicine's life-saving ethic.[107]

A study of nurses' feelings about euthanasia was done at the University of Washington Hospital and Swedish Hospital Medical Center.[108] Findings indicated that nurses heard requests for positive or direct euthanasia from terminally ill patients and their families more frequently than did physicians. The underlying assumption was that nurses have more interaction with the patient and family than does the physician. More nurses were uncomfortable when physicians were not practicing negative euthanasia, "letting the patient die," than when the physician did follow this ethic. Nurses generally demonstrated more desire than physicians for social changes to allow euthanasia, for example, legislation. Eighty-five percent of the nurses surveyed would practice negative euthanasia with a signed statement of consent. This seems to demonstrate that nurses hold the value of the patient's right to maintain control and make decisions about the end of life and way of dying. More nurses than physicians supported the concept of using a committee or board for resolving difficult philosophical decisions about euthanasia.

Nurses may want to consider an alternative to euthanasia in attempting to articulate their own moral ethic of care for the dying. Dyck's proposal of an ethic called benemortasia is that of a happy or good death, but one that is not necessarily painless and/or hastened by physicians' action in order to be "good" for the individual. This ethic was mentioned earlier in the chapter in the section on Euthanasia. According to this ethic, the compassion and freedom of the nurse are increased in relationship with a specific irreversibly ill patient who has the freedom to refuse interventions that only prolong the dying process and with the patient's physician, who has the freedom under this ethic to honor the patient's wishes, for example, choices of how to live while dying.[109] This ethic adheres to the Commandment that thou shalt not kill. Taking a human life is viewed as a wrong-making characteristic of action. The major focus is on preserving the life and values of the human community with mercy and compassion for the individual. A moral distinction is made in this ethic between acts that *permit* death and acts that *cause* death.[110]

Nurses are often involved with patients who are, or are considerd to be, suicidal. Suicide and assisting in suicide are generally considered to be unjustifiable acts of killing.[111] Suicide is viewed as the ultimate way of shutting out all other people from one's life and of saying that life is no longer worthwhile. This stance negates H. Richard Niebuhr's view that lives are shaped by our responses to others and their responses to us, and that this puts us in responsible relation to others. Suicide in any form negates this aspect of human community.[112] One of the corresponding problems with legalization of voluntary euthanasia by the community is that it does, indeed, sanction the physician's assistance in suicide.

In summary, the ethic of benemortasia maintains that (1) the individual's life is not solely at the disposal of that person because he/she is part of a human community; (2) the individual has the freedom to make moral choices; (3) every individual life has some worth; and (4) the supreme value is goodness, in Western religious traditions referred to as God, to which the dying and those who care for the dying are responsible. This involves the good of the individual and the community. No one human being or community can presume to know who should live or die.[113] Dyck suggests that in carrying out this ethic, patients may need advocates other than physicians and nurses.[114] As there may be recognized conflict between the authority and autonomy of the health professionals and that of the patient, the patient needs someone outside of this conflict who represents his interests. Health professionals may adhere to the medical ethic that says one should do every-thing one can to preserve life. Death is seen as the failure of medical tech-nology and knowledge. Again, the question arises as to what is harm for a given patient.

The ethic of benemortasia, the points made by Smith, and the philosophy of the hospice movement provide starting points for discussion within and outside the profession by nurses confronted with a patient and family who want the plug pulled or do not want heroic measures instituted. The Dying Person's Bill of Rights offers another framework for discussions and decision making about ethical issues that arise in care of the dying person, whether an adult or child.[115] The Dying Person's Bill of Rights includes such ideas as rights to treatment as a living human being until death, maintenance of a sense of hopefulness, expression of one's own feelings and emotions about approaching death, participation in decisions concerning one's care, freedom from pain, the right not to die alone, to have one's questions answered honestly without deception, to have help from and for one's family in ac-cepting one's death, to maintain one's individuality, and to be cared for by caring, sensitive, knowledgeable people. The last right, that is to be cared for by caring, sensitive, knowledgeable people, implies that these people, including nurses, have deliberated and continue to consider developments affecting those ethical dilemmas posed by the technologies that may or may not be used to maintain life.

Kluge, a philosopher, proposes two issues that must be settled by society in the face of present confusion over questions of death and dying.[116] These issues have been mentioned in this chapter. One is whether or not there are any absolute moral laws and intrinsic values in this area. If there are, they must be identified, e.g., any life is worthwhile or killing is not allowed. Secondly, with the identification of absolute moral laws and values, one must identify who counts as a person in terms of moral duties and obligations. According to Kluge, one may not be considered a person simply by definition as a human being. Is one a person by virtue of certain functioning, and/or capacity for relationship with others, and/or possession of a certain aware-ness? The critical issue of "humanhood" was previously raised in the writing of the theologian Joseph Fletcher.[117] He developed a "profile of man" with positive and negative criteria for "humanhood." Nurses as health profes-sionals and as members of the human community should be working on these issues at a conscious level with others. No one person or group can settle issues of this magnitude. One might consider using the "ideal observer" concept discussed in Chapter 2 as a framework for consideration of these crucial issues.

To focus primarily on a patient-centered ethic as we have done in this section is not to ignore the hospital and public policy issues that occur around society's priorities for health and illness and allocation of resources, for example. Chapter 10 focuses on some ways that nursing is and can be actively involved in such areas as legislation, where death and dying create ethical dilemmas for health providers, consumers, legislators, and the human community at large. In terms of community, one wonders if nursing has any obligation to those individuals who die alone in the community. Does the community have obligations to these individuals?

Living wills for individuals, hospital guidelines, and legislation are all significant steps in seeking paths to resolving some of the ethical dilemmas that exist today around death and dying. Nurses should, at least, be able to articulate and develop positions on these dilemmas that confront them as individuals and professionals. "Ethical rounds" for nurses, "death and dying" courses in basic nursing education, and continuing education efforts in the area of health care ethics provide forums for doing this within the nursing community and with other health disciplines.

To talk about the dignity and death of one individual is to talk about the life of everyone in the human community.

REFERENCES

1. Kübler-Ross E: On Death and Dying. New York, Macmillan, 1969
2. Glaser BG, Strauss AL: Awareness of Dying. Chicago, Aldine, 1965
3. Brim O et al (eds): The Dying Patient. New York, Russell Sage, 1970
4. Cooper IS: It's Hard to Leave When the Music's Playing. New York, Norton, 1977
5. Mitford J: The American Way of Death. New York, Simon & Schuster, 1963
6. Parsons T: Death in American society: a brief working paper. Am Behav Sci 6:61–65, 1963
7. Gortner SR: Death with dignity: ethical issues in the proposed legislation. ANA Clinical Sessions, 1974. New York, Appleton, 1975, p 169
8. Film: Who Should Survive? Joseph P. Kennedy, Jr. Foundation, 1971
9. Morison RS: Death: process or event? In Steinfels P, Veatch RM (eds): Death Inside Out. The Hastings Center Report. New York, Harper & Row, 1974, p 68
10. Report of the Ad Hoc Committee of the Harvard Medical School to Examine the Definition of Brain Death: A definition of irreversible coma. JAMA 205:85–88, 1968
11. Ibid. pp 85–86
12. Ibid. p 87

13. Kansas Statutes Annotated, c. 77–202, Definition of Death [L. 1970, c. 378, 1; July 1]. Supplementary Pocket Part, p 45

14. Capron AM: The Quinlan decision: Shifting the burden of decision making. Hastings Cent Rep February 1976, p 17

15. Matter of Quinlan, 70 NJ 10 (1976), 355 A2d 647 (NJ 1976)

16. Kass LR: Death as an event. In Steinfels P, Veatch RM (eds): op cit, pp 71–80

17. Ramsey P: The indignity of "Death with Dignity." In Steinfels P, Veatch RM: op cit, pp 81–96

18. Morison RS: op cit, pp 65–67

19. Ibid: p 66

20. Ibid: p 66

21. Ibid: p 69

22. Ibid: p 69

23. Kass LR: op cit, p 73

24. Ibid: p 78

25. Bok S: Lecture on severely defective newborns given in Ethics and Decision Making in Medicine, Harvard Medical School, January 19, 1977

26. Ibid: January 19, 1977

27. Duff RS, Campbell AGM: Moral and ethical dilemmas in the special-care nursery. N Engl J Med 289:890–94, 1973

28. McCormick RA: To save or let die: the dilemma of modern medicine. JAMA 229:172–76, 1974

29. Shaw A: Dilemmas of "informed consent" in children. N Engl J Med 289:885–90, 1973

30. Ramsey P: The Patient as Person. New Haven and London, Yale University Press, 1970, pp 122–23

31. Brody H: Ethical Decisions in Medicine. Boston, Little, Brown, 1976, p 72

32. Fried C: Terminating life support: out of the closet! N Engl J Med 295:390, 1976

33. Brody H: op cit, p 72

34. Ufema JK: Dare to care for the dying. Am J Nurs 76:89, 1976

35. Simons SM: The obligation to live vs. the option to die. South Med J 65:731, 1972

36. Branson R, Casebeer K: The Quinlan decision: obscuring the role of the physician. Hastings Cent Rep February 1976, p 9

37. Ibid: p 9

38. Ibid: p 9

39. Heifetz MS, Magel C: The Right to Die. New York, Putnam, 1975

40. Fletcher GP: Legal aspects of the decision not to prolong life. JAMA 203:120, 1968

41. Fletcher J: Ethics and euthanasia. Am J Nurs 73:670, 672, 1973

42. Dyck AJ: Beneficent euthanasia and benemortasia: alternative views of mercy. In Kohl M (ed): Beneficent Euthanasia. Buffalo, New York, Prometheus, 1975, p 120

43. Fletcher J: op cit, p 671
44. Mansson HH: Justifying the final solution. Omega 3:79-87, May, 1972
45. Rawls J: A Theory of Justice. Cambridge, Harvard University Press, 1971, pp 131-35
46. Dyck AJ: op cit, pp 124-26
47. Weber LJ: Ethics and euthanasia: another view. Am J Nurs 73:1228-1230, 1973
48. Kamisar Y: From Euthanasia legislation: Some nonreligious objections. In Gorovitz S et al (eds): Moral Problems in Medicine. Englewood Cliffs, NJ, Prentice-Hall, 1976, p 402
49. Brody H: op cit, p 195
50. Heifetz MD: op cit, pp 111-12
51. Weber LJ: op cit, p 1231
52. White RB: Case studies in Bioethics: A demand to die. Hastings Cent Rep June 1975, pp 9-10
53. Reich W: The physician's "duty" to preserve life. Hastings Cent Rep, April 1975, p 15
54. Weber LJ: op cit, pp 1229-31
55. Pontoppidan H: Optimum care for hopelessly ill patients. N Engl J Med 295:362-64, 1976
56. Rabkin MT, Gillerman G, Rice NR: Orders not to resuscitate. N Engl J Med 295:364-66, 1976
57. A Living Will: Prepared and distributed by Euthanasia Educational Council, 250 West 57 Street, New York, NY 10019
58. Bok S: Personal directions for care at the end of life. N Engl J Med 295:368-69, 1976
59. Garland M: The right to die in California: politics, legislation, and natural death. Hastings Cent Rep, October 1976, p 5
60. Ramsey P: op cit, p 198
61. Duff RS, Campbell AGM: op cit, pp 890-94
62. Shaw A: op cit, pp 885-90
63. Kluge EHW: The Practice of Death. New Haven and London, Yale University Press, 1975, pp 182-209
64. Zachary RB: Ethical and social aspects of treatment of spina bifida. In Gorovits S et al (eds): Moral Problems in Medicine. Englewood Cliffs, NJ, Prentice-Hall, 1976, pp 342-52
65. Freeman JM: Is there a right to die—quickly? In Gorovitz S et al (eds): op cit, pp 354-56
66. Engelhardt T Jr: Aiding the death of young children. In Kohl M (ed): op cit, pp 180-92
67. Heifetz MD: op cit, p 81
68. Kant I: Duties towards the body in regard to life. In Gorovitz S et al (eds): op cit, pp 376-77
69. Heifetz MD: op cit, p 79
70. Williams G: From The right to commit suicide. In Gorovitz S et al (eds): op cit, p 388
71. Heifetz MD: op cit, p 79

72. Murphey GE: Suicide and the right to die. In Gorovitz S et al (eds): op cit, pp 387–88
73. Rockwell DA, O'Brien W: Physicians' knowledge and attitudes about suicide. JAMA 225:1347–49, 1973
74. Heifetz MD: op cit, p 96
75. Ibid: p 81
76. Berger P, Hamburg B, Hamburg D: Mental health: progress and problems. Daedalus, Winter 1977, p 270
77. Murphy GE: op cit, pp 387–88
78. Hook S: The ethics of suicide. In Kohl M (ed): op cit, pp 60–63
79. Ibid: pp 66–67
80. Gortner SR: op cit, p 169
81. Lester D, Getty C, Kneisl CR: Attitudes of nursing students and nursing faculty toward death. Nurs Res 23:50–59, 1974
82. Caughill RE (ed): The Dying Patient: A Supportive Approach. Boston, Little, Brown, 1976
83. Griffin JJ: Family decision: a crucial factor in terminating life. Am J Nurs 75:794–96, 1975
84. Schorr TM: Editorial: the right to die. Am J Nurs 76:53, 1976
85. Strauss AL, Glaser BG: Anguish: A Case History of a Dying Trajectory. Mill Valley, California, Sociology Press, 1970
86. Quint JC: The Nurse and the Dying Patient. New York, Macmillan, 1967
87. ——: The threat of death—some consequences for patients and nurses. Nurs Forum 8:287–300, 1969
88. Yeaworth RC, Kapp FT, Winget C: Attitudes of nursing students toward the dying patient. Nurs Res 23:20–24, 1974
89. Kuhn ME: Death and dying: the right to live—the right to die. ANA Clinical Sessions—1974. New York, Appleton, 1975, pp 184–89
90. Hershey N: On the question of prolonging life. Am J Nurs 71:521–22, 1971
91. Beauchamp JA: Euthanasia and the nurse practitioner. Nurs Forum 14:57, 1975
92. Rabkin MT, et al: op cit, p 365
93. Ibid: p 366
94. Assell RA: If you were dying. In Caughill RE (ed): The Dying Patient: A Supportive Approach. Boston, Little, Brown, 1976, pp 47–71
95. Gartner CR: Growing up to dying: the child, the parents, and the nurse. In Caughill RE (ed): The Dying Patient: A Supportive Approach. Boston, Little, Brown, 1976, pp 159–89
96. Hampe S: Needs of the grieving spouse in a hospital setting. Nurs Res 24:116–17, 1975
97. Michaels DR: Too much in need of support to give any? Nurs Res 21:286, 1972
98. Strank RA: Caring for the chronic sick and dying: a study of attitudes. Nurs Times 68:166–69, 1972

99. Gortner SR: op cit, p 175
100. Smith DH: Some ethical considerations in caring for the dying. ANA Clinical Sessions—1974. New York, Appleton, 1975, pp 177–78
101. Ibid: p 181
102. Ramsey P: op cit, pp 116–17
103. Frankena WK: Ethics, 2nd ed. Englewood Cliffs, NJ, Prentice-Hall, 1973, pp 45–52
104. Smith DH: op cit, pp 180–81
105. Ramsey P: op cit, p. 153
106. Wentzel KB: The dying are the living. Am J Nurs 76:956–57, 1976
107. Ramsey P: op cit, p 164
108. Brown NK, Donovan JT, Bulger RJ, Laws EH: How do nurses feel about euthanasia and abortion? Am J Nurs 71:1415–16, 1971
109. Dyck AJ: An alternative to the ethic of euthanasia. In Williams RH (ed): To Live and to Die: When, Why, and How. New York, Springer, 1974, pp 102–4
110. Ibid: p 104
111. Ibid: p 104
112. Ibid: pp 106, 111
113. Ibid: p 111
114. Ibid: p 109
115. Barbus AJ: The dying person's bill of rights. Am J Nurs 75:99, 1975
116. Kluge EHK: op cit, pp 243–44
117. Fletcher J: Indicators of humanhood: A tentative profile of man. Hastings Cent Rep, November 1972, pp 1–4

8

BEHAVIOR CONTROL

INTRODUCTION

The long history of social evolution has engaged the human species in an endless struggle to understand, predict, influence, and control human behavior. The notion of the common good has been invoked in most instances for coercing an individual to conform to social mores. Historically, the tyranny of the majority has had limited results, especially in private life, since the machinery of repression has had no efficient ways to cope with the deviance and nonconformity engaged in within the confines of one's own home and in one's private relationships. Laws, developed to deal with this area of life, to a large extent functioned more as expressions of public morality than as incursions on private liberty. However, recently developed control methods make it possible now to exact conformity with greater reliability and less potential for resistance than has been the case in the past. Increasingly, we have the technology to effectively engineer consent, which can thereby eliminate personal license and still leave individuals with the feeling that they are free. This situation may appeal as a therapeutic tool to those who work with the "hard-core" criminal or the severely mentally ill; however, such developments in behavior control, with widespread use, can also serve to unhinge the conventional political morality basic to modern democracy. The basic ethical problem of behavior control arises in the dilemma of how to maintain personal liberty in situations where its suppression can be rationalized not only by the common welfare but also by the individual's happiness.[1]

The potential success of behavior control techniques to change people—prison inmates, mental patients, and the entire gamut of people seeking psychiatric help with the goal of self-fulfillment and self-realization—has become the source of controversy within the larger debate as to society's proper response to deviant behavior. The concept of unintended consequences, which maintains that reforms and innovations often carry with them effects of a social nature contrary to the stated purpose of the intended goals, becomes a central concern in developing techniques to control behavior.[2] For example, according to sociologists and social historians, the original intent in establishing asylums for the mentally ill, which was to provide a protective setting with treatment and human conditions, also had the unintentional consequences of turning them into warehouses for the mentally ill where loss of individuality, depersonalization, and dehumanization resulted.[3-5] The concerns surrounding behavior control and the unintended consequences can be understood in the context of the three social dilemmas that prisons and mental hospitals share: (1) How does the institutional social structure affect attempts at treatment and rehabilitation? (2) How can these institutions meet both the demands of society and the needs of the individuals they serve? (3) What kind of control should be exercised over the development and application of behavior control techniques?[6] Although the criminal justice system and the mental health system both utilize forms of behavior control, this chapter will focus, in the main, on the latter.

During the past 20 years, we have come to recognize that prisons and mental hospitals fall far short of meeting the goals set for them by society. Critics, both in and out of the mental health field, traced this failure to a number of variables, including the basic factor that the social structure of these institutions not only did not always support their stated goals but at times tended to undermine their purpose.[7-10] The recognition of these problems led to three changes that affected the "total institution" nature of the mental hospital. As an attempt to alter the social structure of mental hospitals, Jones developed the therapeutic community concept in the United Kingdom, which became a major reform movement during the 1950s and 1960s.[11,12] The second change, the community mental health movement, arose from an awareness of the negative aspects of maintaining a patient in a total institution over a long period of time. This change resulted in a shift away from almost total reliance on public institutions with their involuntary incarceration and treatment to a more voluntaristic and pluralistic system.

The third change, which made the first two possible, has been the development of behavior control technology, all of which has become more sophisticated, more effective, and more efficient. This technology includes psychotropic drugs, electroshock therapy, psychosurgery, behavior modification, and other psychological techniques. This fundamental change, developments in technology, has raised basic legal and ethical questions regarding the rights of patients and the role of staff in a situation where some view psychiatric personnel as double agents, that is, a regulatory agent for the state and a therapeutic agent for the patient. This can, and does, create a conflict-of-interest problem.[13,14]

Before proceeding to a more detailed discussion of specific forms of behavior control, it will be helpful to define the term itself and to consider the fundamental problems of deviancy and coercion. London defined behavior control as getting people to do someone else's bidding such as has been depicted in several popular books.[15,16-19] In the broadest sense, behavior control can be understood as a special form of behavioral change. For example, in a psychiatric setting, treatment offered to or imposed on a patient to a large extent may be designed to satisfy the wishes of others. Behavioral change that satisfies others, the community or society, for example, may or may not satisfy the patient's wishes to change.[20] The use of behavior control with the mentally ill has been questioned on the grounds that such treatment deprives patients of the fundamental right to choose their course of action.[21-23] As behavior control technology develops and becomes more available, and as the psychiatric categories seem to expand to include more attitudes and behaviors defined as deviant, at least one critic fears a conspiracy to establish a so-called therapeutic state.[24] Preventive psychiatry continues to define more and more problems of human behavior as falling within its jurisdiction, yet the critics maintain that its practitioners are unable to cope with its present scope. This inability to deliver the goods, so to speak, may be considered as both an ethical problem and safeguard against unchecked power.

DEVIANCY AND MENTAL ILLNESS

Every society has its rules and social norms. It is generally expected in a given society that a majority of the people will conform to these rules and norms most of the time. Additionally, every society has its nonconformists, who may be artists with their bohemian lifestyle, that most communities within society will tolerate without attempting to control as long as such a lifestyle does not deviate too much, from the established norm. The nonconformists, usually considered as deviants and social problems in our society, do not constitute a homogeneous group, and the characteristics that bring them societal attention do not lend themselves to easy classification. Generally speaking, the most obvious groups considered deviant in our own society fall into the following, nonexclusive, categories: medical (the mentally ill); intellectual (the mentally retarded); chronologic (the senile); social (the alcoholic); economic (other drug abusers); sexual (the homosexual); or doctrinal nonconformity (the sociopolitical radical). These groups share two things in common. First, their behavior is proscribed or controlled by law, and second, society increasingly seeks them out for "treatment" instead of "punishment."[25] Basically, social groups create deviance when they make rules whose infraction constitutes deviance and when they apply those rules to particular individuals and label them as outsiders. It follows then that deviance is not a quality of the act the person commits, but rather a consequence of the application by others of rules and sanctions to a so-called offender. The deviant person is one to whom that label has successfully been applied and deviant behavior is behavior that people so label.[26]

Those persons whom we call mentally ill tend to be at variance with the mores and conventions of society. The fact that this condition usually has behavioral, rather than with physiological symptoms alone, casts those so labeled into the role of the social deviant. Mental illness is not easy to define or to determine, and this situation becomes compounded by the fact that different societies may have different tolerance levels for the sort of deviation that becomes labeled as mental illness.

The concept, dangerousness, has been the paramount consideration in the legal commitment procedure within our mental health system. That means that for the mentally ill deviant, the only legitimate justification for civil commitment was thought to be a provable likelihood of dangerous acts toward the self or toward others. However, the mental health field does not possess the tools to determine, with any degree of precision, those who will be dangerous. Dangerousness, like any number of other things including beauty, is, to some extent, in the eye of the beholder. Although the general public has tended to associate dangerousness with mental illness, the American Psychiatric Association has indicated that about ten percent of the hospitalized mentally ill can be considered dangerous.[27,28] However, according to other sources, this figure of ten percent may be grossly inflated. The base rate of violent behavior (except for suicide) by those labeled mentally ill is no different than for the general population.[29]

Numerous experts have pointed to the inadequacy of the criteria for predicting who will commit a dangerous act.[30-33] One critique of the predictive techniques emphasizes that violent behavior is not only a function of personality but also a function of social context. This provides one explanation as to why the traditional psychiatric approach, which emphasizes personality, would have limited predictive value.[34] The above comments are not intended to imply that no traditional psychiatric clues are valid; only that such validity has yet to be established. The difficulty involved in predicting dangerousness increases when the patient has never actually performed an assaultive act. This problem obviously becomes particularly relevant to involuntary hospitalization situations. Some believe that mental health professionals, since they have no reliable criteria, tend to over predict dangerousness. In such instances, so the argument goes, these professionals have stereotyped ideas of the personality attributes of dangerous individuals that have no valid relationship to the occurrence of dangerous acts. Rather, they commit themselves to these stereotypes because of theoretical constructs that cause them to attend selectively to certain data.[35] In addition to the problems of identification and prediction of dangerous behavior, some, including the National Council on Crime and Delinquency, maintain that neither mental hospitals nor prisons are now capable of treating persons labeled as dangerous. It must be seen as a bizarre system of criminal justice that confines mostly those who cannot be identified as dangerous, and equally bizarre a mental health system that commits mostly those who cannot be treated.

COERCION AND FREEDOM

The following comments come from an essay by William Gaylin, a psychoanalyst.[36] He points out that in the United States freedom constitutes a dominant value; however, the structure of organized society depends on defined limits of freedom. The legal system supplies the definitions of permissible behavior and also establishes the coercion force that society may use to insure compliance. Therefore, coercion may not necessarily always be an evil. The basis of civilization depends to a great extent on the right of the state to coerce its citizens. These statements lead to the realization that we must weigh society's right to coerce against the individual's right to freedom. Furthermore, one needs to think through what constitutes a coerced, as distinguished from a free, act. Freedom, a principle to which psychiatry aspires rather than a concept that it often employs, has not been incorporated to any extent into a theory of behavior, since it has difficulty fitting freedom with theory that tends toward a deterministic view. With a frame of reference that defines man as less than rational and motivated more by appeals to emotions than to reason, psychiatry, and especially psychoanalysis, is far more comfortable with the concept of coercion.

Since those things that people experience are the true determinants of behavior, the perception of danger becomes the crucial issue in coercion. To understand coercion one must understand that which threatens man. The problem is not so much the coercion involved in physical force and threatening survival itself, but survival equivalents such as threat of isolation, loss of love, social humiliation, and so on.

As stated earlier, the social order relies to some extent on the right to coercion. Along with the legal dimensions of coercion, society has also given a moral privilege to coercion when such action is done in the individual's best interest. For example, certain parental behavior coerces children, but society permits this because of the assumption that parents have the child's best interest at heart. Also, in the field of health, coercion has a traditional respectability and legal sanction, and psychiatry, as a branch of medicine, has engaged in coercion. Indeed, one might correctly say that, in the recent past, the abrogation of the legal rights of the mentally ill, the denial of due process, the confinement beyond the limits the law tolerates for criminals represent a gross example of coercion.

Behavior control represents a broad spectrum of activities, including psychiatric therapy, political propaganda, commercial advertising, religious and moral education, and rehabilitation of deviant persons. The major categories of behavior control in the mental health field that will be discussed in this chapter are psychotherapy, psychosurgery, and psychopharmacology. Practitioners in the field readily accept the fact that patients should be protected from outright coercion, and this belief has been formalized in statutes and regulations. The idea that the patient should also be protected from more subtle pressures is not only more difficult for many mental health professionals to accept, but also the problems of such regulation become more difficult as well.[37]

PSYCHOTHERAPY

Psychotherapy has gone through three developmental stages during the twentieth century. The argument has been made that each of these stages has been in response to the psychosocial motif dominating the society at that time.[38] Stage One came into being with the development of psychoanalysis. This occurred around the beginning of this century when Freud and Breuer first published their works and formed the Psychoanalytic Society in 1902. Essentially, psychoanalysis treats by uncovering and exposing unconscious material that had been repressed. The patients, mostly middle-class women, lived in the Victorian era of Vienna, known for its standards of proper behavior and repression of sexuality. Psychoanalysis came into being in this era to deal with its major psychosocial motif. A number of factors converged and other psychotherapeutic schools developed with their own theories and techniques. One problem with all psychotherapeutic approaches involved in long-term therapy has been identified as the lack of evidence to prove its effectiveness for patients. The fact remains that traditional psychodynamic therapies have not produced empirical validation of the treatment efficacy. Two problems arise in the attempt to research this area. The first problem is defining what is to be measured, which rests on the larger problem of the definition of normal or healthy. The second problem arises regarding methodology or ways of evaluating possible long-range effects from psychotherapy on both individuals and on society as a whole. Psychotherapy, of any type, can occur between a middle-class patient and therapist who share more or less similar attitudes and values and this process may be a voluntary activity chosen by the patient. However, it can also occur as an involuntary activity when the patient, who may or may not share values and attitudes with the therapist, becomes legally committed. Therapy has been viewed as a political act in either case, in that the therapist can encourage patients to either adjust to or rebel against their environment. However, the potential for using psychotherapy as a coercive tool of social control increases in the situation of involuntary commitment. Psychotherapy can be based on the social and economic biases of the therapist rather than the patient's behavior, and as such can become a coercive tool operating mainly on those very groups who are most helpless to change the social context in which their problems arise.[39]

Stage Two occurred during the 1950s and 1960s with the development of psychotherapy based on principles of conditioning. The generalized term behavior modification became the generic name for those methods emphasizing a behavioristic orientation. Another activist treatment, crisis intervention, lead to the establishment of crisis intervention centers where clients could come in or telephone at any time in an attempt to deal with their problems. These two approaches shared several things: direct attack on the symptoms presented, without going into the underlying cause, short duration of therapy, and the possibility of a more technologic basis for therapy than had been available in previous therapeutic approaches. Stage Two represents a shift away from treating causes to an era of treatment geared toward symptom relief.

Stage Three grew out of the affluence and leisure that the large middle-class had achieved in the late 1960s and early 1970s, when society passed from the age of anxiety to the age of ennui. The overriding preoccupation for many became the achievement of value and meaning in life. Psychotherapy shifted away from a focus on the relief of discomfort and pain to meeting the demands of the populace who sought a richer life with deeper experiences and relationships. At present, the developments from all three stages continue to function to meet the different needs of a vast number of individuals with a great variety of reasons for seeking help or having it imposed on them. As indicated for Stage One, the developments in Stages Two and Three, separately or in combination, can also serve as coercive tools of social control.

Behavior control, as a potential ethical dilemma, varies with the different methods of treatment utilized. Psychotherapy has been widely accepted and practiced as the major means that therapists had to deal with psychologic disorders. It has been less recognized or discussed as a means of controlling people. Long-term insight therapy can be utilized systematically to influence attitudes and values, if not overt behavior, toward conventional norms of conduct. One could make the argument, however, that because this therapy method is slow, technologically benign, and limited to a relatively small target population, the risks incurred, as far as behavior control goes, are few. As behavior changes occur, the patient develops an accompanying increase in his awareness, enabling him to monitor his own behavior changes to some extent. Furthermore, to a large degree, clients participating in insight therapy remain outside the large mental hospitals, so that the factors of institutional social structure do not affect the attempt at treatment and rehabilitation.

Stage Two, with its principles of conditioning, deserves more attention, since such treatment techniques have been rigorously criticized as being repressive and dehumanizing. In the light of such criticism, Ervin, aware of the ethical problems in behavior control, makes the point that our fascination with technology leads us to overrate the promise as well as the threat of these new techniques.[40] Such techniques received attention in the controversial film of Anthony Burgess' novel, *Clockwork Orange*,[41] Generally speaking, that type of behavior control referred to as behavior therapy or behavior modification is one in which the therapist manipulates the environment and the consequences of a person's behavior in order to change that behavior. The therapist reinforces desired behavior while the behavior not wanted receives an adverse response, or, at a minimum, receives no reward. Ivar Lovaas' work with autistic children who had not been reached by normal methods of love, compassion, and punishment provides us with an example of behavior modification. The therapist placed barefoot autistic children into a room with a metal grid in the floor. The children periodically received an electric shock that they could avoid only by throwing themselves into the arms of an adult. After a time, these children began to seek out adults on their own without the shock. Another example involved a young boy who had been strapped to his bed for more than seven years. When he was not strapped to the bed, he would take bites out of his shoulder. After three severe electrical jolts with a cattle prod, he stopped the biting behavior. However, upon return to his usual ward, he reverted to his previous behavior. The physician visited the ward and discovered that as soon as the boy tried to bite himself, the nurses would immediately run up and lovingly hug him, thereby rewarding his abnormal biting behavior. Such behavior modification techniques as described here may seem, and indeed may be, cruel. Yet in the second example, the case of misapplied love maintained a situation that also could be viewed as cruel.[42]

Success using this type of therapy has been rather limited, since the major difficulty of having changed behavior persisting over time remains. However, the success obtained in the treatment of chronic patients has been accomplished with behavioral techniques.[43] The larger question that arises has to do with the possible gains as against the possible losses. Considerable evidence that people's behavior can be programmed fairly easily now exists. One basic premise underlying much current research seems to be that man is after all an animal, and many features of his learning and behavior share similarities with those found in a large number of animals. The argument goes that it should be possible to train a human by the same methods that have been so well developed for animals—rats, dogs, and pigeons, for example. In general, behavior therapy and behavior modification methods have been shown to be somewhat superior to other forms of therapy; however, difficult disorders do not produce very positive results and no evidence shows that the effects persist over time.[44] These comments must be taken with the realization that most, if not all, psychotherapeutic techniques have limitations, so alternatives may or may not exist. One study concluded that traditional methods of treating hospitalized psychiatric patients, including individual therapy, group therapy, work therapy, and drug therapy, do not affect differentially the discharged patients' community functioning as measured by recidivism and post-hospital employment.[45] But in recent years, with the development of community mental health programs, many patients receive treatment outside hospitals. However, this development has not solved the baffling problems of major mental illness. These programs' major techniques, individual and group therapy, have had, at best, limited effectiveness and they either do not reach, or are inimical to, major segments of the population requiring help.[46,47] In short, any criticism of behavior therapy must take into account the ethical dilemmas involved, but also the state of the science and art of psychiatry. This entire situation has been made more acute by the fact that in formulating new rules of mental health, the professionals have created new classes of mentally ill individuals to the extent that we possibly have a contemporary exaggeration of the concept of mental illness.[48]

This more recently developed type of therapy, behavior modification, has been greatly influenced by Skinnerian behaviorism with its emphasis on environmental control and shaping of behavior.[49,50] The antibehaviorism viewpoint expressed in the writings of Carl Rogers and others, including Jourard, contend that while the so-called behavioristic approach to psychiatry acknowledges an individual's susceptibility to manipulation by another, it also ignores the possible deleterious impact of this manipulation on the whole person and, additionally, on the manipulator himself.[51-53] They believe that the essential factor in the psychotherapeutic encounter is an honest, loving, spontaneous relationship between the therapist and patient.[54,55] On the other hand, a behavioristic point of view could make the argument that apparent spontaneity on the therapist's part can well be the most effective means of manipulating the patient's behavior. The therapist has been programmed by his training into a fairly effective behavior control machine of sorts, and most likely this machine is most effective when it appears least like a machine. To summarize this point, a science of psychology or psychiatry seeks to determine the lawful relationships in behavior, while the science of behavior control rests on the assumption that these relationships are to be used to deliberately influence, control, or change behavior. This orientation implies a controller who has an ethical and value system.[56] However, the reciprocity of the relationship between the controller and the controlled, an important facet of behavior control, often goes overlooked.

PSYCHOSURGERY

Psychosurgery, or surgery to alter behavior, has become a topic of discussion in scientific literature, congressional reports, legal documents, and in lay publications. The general term, psychosurgery, refers to a number of surgical procedures such as cingulotomy, amygdalatomy, thalamotomy, lobotomy, and lobectomy. In 1970, a neurosurgeon and a psychiatrist wrote a book entitled *Violence and the Brain* that detailed the application of neurosurgery techniques to the problems of violent behavior.[57] The response to this book vividly underscored the growing concern with the social role of such experts who have within their power, along with the geneticist, the possibility of turning the classic philosophical question, "What is man?" to a very different question, "What kind of man are we going to construct?"[58-63,64] In turn, and in reaction to the response, Vernon Mark, a neurosurgeon, along with Robert Neville, a philosopher, offered some reflections about the social issues involved in psychosurgery by making the point that most criticisms either construe this type of surgery as capable of more than it can deliver or assume that such surgery would be appropriate to use for purposes of control in those instances when no surgeon would agree to such a use.[65] Psychosurgery, like any other technology, can be misused; nevertheless, the basic problem stems from the dichotomy in basic approaches to behavior.

    Many social scientists, and others in the mental health field, view certain behavioral abnormalities, such as aggressive, assaultive behavior or intractable depression, as resulting from unusual or abnormal environmental stress and that brain function or dysfunction does not play a part in abnormal behavior.

Obviously, no human behavior, normal or abnormal, can be the consequence of the brain alone without the environment and, obviously, no behavior, whatever its environmental determinants, occurs without the brain freighting its mechanical impulses with emotion and culture. A statement that recognizes the brain's involvement in behavior does not lead to the conclusion, as some critics think, that all behavior should be controlled through the brain.

Mark and Neville continue by developing three alternative defenses of psychosurgical procedures, which illustrate their thesis regarding the appropriateness of this type of behavior control. Importantly, they reject the first two alternatives. Alternative one states that medical means should be undertaken to improve any behavior, normal or abnormal, whenever possible. This position has the advantage of avoiding the difficult task of defining normality and the disadvantage of making medicine the authority on improvement of what constitutes the good life and the proper means of achieving it. Alternative two states that any undesirable, abnormal behavior should be treated by whatever medical means available, including psychosurgery, if it can be shown to be the most efficient method with the least risks. Two problems arise with this position. First, psychiatric neurosurgery, despite great technical advances, is still experimental and irreversible. The second problem, that a person will be set up for psychosurgery simply because someone else does not desire his behavior, received a dramatic treatment in the book and film, *One Flew Over the Cuckoo's Nest*.[66] Alternative three, accepted by Mark and Neville, states that drastic procedures such as psychosurgery should be used only when behavior is abnormal and "bad," primarily because of a brain abnormality. Then any abnormal behavior not associated with brain disease will be dealt with by political and social means, not medical ones.

The point must be made before leaving this topic that environmental cues controlled the German population to the extent that many, if not most, played at least a passive part in one of the worst scenes of carnage ever enacted on the human stage. Some would argue that the human personality and brain, programmed specifically for environmental inputs and controls, receives its most outstanding threat for behavior control from that which already exists and not from psychosurgery or drugs.

PSYCHOPHARMACOLOGY

Several writers have dealt with both the pharmacological developments potentially enabling us to control human emotions and mental functioning as well as the extent of drug use in this country.[67-70] At one time, we commonly thought of psychotropic drugs mainly for use with patients diagnosed as psychotic or depressed. More recently, it has been documented that increasingly relatively normal people use these agents in order to cope with the stresses encountered in daily life. Statistics indicate that the production and distribution of psychotropic drugs have become a major component of the drug industry. In 1967 estimates of 180 million prescriptions for these drugs at a cost of 700 million dollars give us some idea of the magnitude of the situation. Data from one study conducted in California indicate that approximately seventeen percent of adults reported frequent use of psychotropic drugs with the figure being twice as high for females as for men and with the heaviest use occurring in the 40-59 age group.[71]

Psychopharmacology emerged as a separate branch within pharmacology after World War II with the discovery of LSD in 1943 and Chlorpromazine in 1952. During the next few years, and with great rapidity, dozens of new compounds became available. Klerman divides psychotropic drugs into three categories depending on the purpose for which they are used, including: (1) drugs used as therapeutic agents for the treatment of psychiatric disorders; (2) drugs used for nontherapeutic purposes, such as recreation or personal enjoyment; and (3) drugs used to enhance performance and capabilities.[72] Ethical issues arise in each category, including that of coercion, which can be a special problem in category one. However, some authorities, pointing to what they call the decentralized character of drug taking, the necessity for repeated doses, and the fact that often pills are self-administered, view the problem of behavior control through drugs as less of an issue than of getting people not to take these drugs.[73] Of all the techniques that modern technology has developed and that can be used for controlling behavior, drugs are certainly among the most widely disseminated and readily available.[74] In a drug culture, where many, if not most, people think a visit to the doctor's office or clinic has been a waste of time unless they come away with some pills and where the medical professional usually reinforces this attitude, the possibility of drug abuse of all kinds, including behavior control, can pose the single most difficult problem for reasons of availability, accessibility, and the general cultural attitude toward drugs.

ETHICAL DILEMMAS

The right to receive treatment and the right to refuse treatment in general and the right to consent to or decline behavior modification techniques in particular raise conflict-of-interest questions. Does the therapist satisfy his own interest or those of the patients, or most likely some combination of the two? In some situations, the therapist serves a third party and this can be a problem, especially when he is an employee of an institution whose interests do not necessarily coincide with the interests of the patient. Third parties often apply subtle, and sometimes not so subtle, pressures that therapists may not be fully aware of or understand. Conflict-of-interest represents one facet of the wider problem of what values, especially what conflicting values, are served by the mental health field. One major obstacle to a greater awareness of these value conflicts comes from the fact that mental health professionals have a marked tendency to assume that they function in a value-free frame of reference. Keenly aware of the patient's conflicts, they may be less inclined to see the conflicts of their own social role. The fact remains that, regardless of theoretical orientation, these professionals are often a party to such conflict.

The larger ethical question involved in behavior control of any type turns on the problem of personal integrity. The essential question then is, "Does the individual have an inviolable, indefeasible, absolute right to be himself, whatever or whoever he is, the product of whatever heredity and environment is his lot, even if he is deviant or dangerous to himself or others?" A whole host of questions for consideration in discussing behavior control include: if the individual is dangerous to himself, does society have the right to intervene to stop him from hurting or destroying himself? Does society have the right or obligation to protect its members from themselves or from others? On what moral ground can it be determined where the limits of individual rights become outweighed by societal rights? Who will decide who is dangerous and on what knowledge base? How is normalcy to be defined for therapy? If a social deviant receives psychiatric treatment, should the aim of that treatment be adjustment or adaptation? Are there ethical grounds for rejecting some or all of the more potent behavior control techniques, even if they prove to be quite effective? When are possible risks from such procedures justified? How is consent obtained and from whom? Is experimentation justified outside of the context of a reasonable belief that the procedure will be therapeutic for the individual? If therapists increasingly use these techniques, should there be some type of regulation device over and beyond informed consent? With regard to this last question, Halleck proposes that any treatment recommendation, for the civilly committed, disturbed patients who have not consented, which involve brain surgery, electric shock therapy, prolonged use of drugs, or behavior therapy, should be reviewed and approved by a monitoring agency.[75] Who will be on this monitoring agency and who will select them? Other questions are: Should such treatment as long-term use of psychotropic drugs or psychosurgery be considered for children? If so, which children will be eligible for this treatment and who will decide on what grounds? Is it ethical to deny such treatment to adults or children if all other treatment approaches have failed? Should such a technique as brain surgery be used as a means to control violent behavior, even if it is of unknown etiology? How does any one of these behavior control techniques determine the relationship between the patient and his doctor, nurse, or family? How does the technology affect the distribution of monetary and other resources for medical care? Who pays for such treatment? What are the possible potential implications of behavior control?

Essentially, the ethical questions boil down to: What kind of behavior should be controlled? Whose behavior is controlled? Who controls? Who decides who controls? How does behavior control affect dignity and freedom? What are the costs of gaining self-control? What social interests justify social control? What instruments of control are warranted to serve the interest of society?[76] All of these questions evolve from several ethical dilemmas involved in behavior control. The dilemma of personal integrity versus society's obligation to protect its members remains perhaps the most central dilemma. The dilemma of immunity versus forfeiture of rights raises the question of what rights to the privacy and inviolability of body and mind should a person lose once he has been diagnosed as mentally ill, especially if he is committed to an institution. The dilemma of procedural rights is concerned with what rights does a patient have to the procedural protection of the suspension, waiver, or forfeiture of these basic rights? The dilemma of rights and goods concerns the possible conflict between the person's right to be different and his potential desire to be free from any misery which his deviance causes. The dilemma of informed voluntary consent raised the problems of mental status and legal status as inhibitions to obtaining informed consent. The dilemma of paternalism and authoritarianism raised the questions that John Stuart Mill addressed. What are the limits on the use of coercion, on the kinds of coercion, and/or the actions coercively prevented or elicited, that one person may use on another in the name of the latter's own good? The fact that the intention of those using the techniques of intervention may be therapeutic does not alter either the paternalistic or authoritarian character of such use under certain circumstances. The dilemma of deceptive labeling concerns the issue of when does enforced treatment, especially that involving irreversible effects, become primitive control under a false therapeutic label?[77]

Kittrie has developed a Therapeutic Bill of Rights because he believes that the philosophical origins of therapeutic programs combined humanism, paternalism, and utilitarian determinism in promoting the public's interest in social defense. The general principles of the Therapeutic Bill of Rights are:

1. No person shall be compelled to undergo treatment except for the defense of society.
2. Man's innate right to remain free of excessive forms of human modification shall be inviolable.

3. No social sanctions may be invoked unless the person subjected to treatment has demonstrated a clear and present danger through truly harmful behavior which is immediately forthcoming or has already occurred.

4. No person shall be subjected to involuntary incarceration or treatment on the basis of a finding of a general condition of status alone. Nor shall the mere conviction for a crime or a finding of not guilty by reason of insanity suffice to have a person automatically committed or treated.

5. No social sanctions whether designated criminal, civil, or therapeutic may be invoked in the absence of the previous right to a judicial or other independent hearing, appointed counsel, and an opportunity to confront those testifying about one's past conduct or therapeutic needs.

6. Dual interference by both the criminal and the therapeutic process is prohibited.

7. An involuntary patient shall have the right to receive treatment.

8. Any compulsory treatment must be the least required reasonably to protect society.

9. All committed persons should have direct access to appointed counsel and the right, without any interference, to petition the courts for relief.

10. Those submitting to voluntary treatment should be guaranteed that they will not be subsequently transferred to a compulsory program through administrative action.[78]

IMPLICATIONS FOR NURSING PRACTICE

The nurse's role in psychiatric settings ranges from custodial keeper-of-the-keys to skilled therapeutic agent. In any of these roles, the nurse has the power to influence and determine, in part, the patient's course of treatment since she observes and interacts with him. Nurses in all specialties have such influence, to some extent, but in the mental health field it takes on special significance because the illness is tied to behavioral symptoms. The mental health nurse, like all other members of the staff, has her own attitudes and value system which affect her definitions of mental illness and mental health. These attitudes and values become a factor in encounters with patients. For example, the field of psychiatry has changed, on paper, its concept of homosexuality. The fact remains, however, that mental health workers in this country are members of the larger society, which, for the most part, has had and continues to have deeply ingrained negative attitudes toward homosexuality. Another ingrained attitude that reflects membership in the culture is the double standard of mental health for men and women, and the differences parallel the sex role stereotypes prevalent in our society.[79]

Once a person enters the mental health system as a patient, the nurse becomes a major source of information regarding his behavior. This is especially so in inpatient settings where longer contacts can occur between nurse and patient and where the nursing staff is the only group to work a 24-hour day. Many decisions regarding treatment occur in team meetings, and the nurse affects the discussion by either providing information or withholding it. If she provides information, then what she reports and how she says it influence the perceptions of the patient by others. In one study, pseudopatients gained admission to mental hospitals by saying they heard voices. Once admitted, they found themselves indelibly labeled with the diagnosis of schizrenia, in spite of their subsequent normal behavior. They kept field notes for the research project and the nurses charted that these "patients" engaged in "compulsive writing." Only the other patients suspected that these pseudopatients were not mentally ill, and were there for other reasons. The staff was unable to acknowledge normal behavior within the hospital milieu. In such a setting, staff tends to see pathology more than it sees normal behavior.[80]

Another potential problem with ethical dimensions that adds to the larger problem of behavior control has to do with whether nurses take the patient seriously. Does the diagnosis of mental illness affect our attitudes toward this category of persons in ways that do not allow us to take seriously what the patient says or does? Because someone is "crazy" it may be easier to dismiss them by not putting any stock in what they communicate, since it does not reflect reality. Such an attitude may be supported by the reward system of the institution where the nurse works as an employee. Not being taken seriously also occurs in situations where adults interact with children.

The medical literature discusses the ethical dilemmas arising from a paternalistic attitude that physicians have toward patients. Such an attitude tends to reduce the adult patient to the status of a child and permits the physician to violate the patient's rights, such as the right to participate in the decision-making process that influences his own welfare. Paternalism is interfering with a person's liberty of action justified by reasons referring exclusively to the welfare, good, happiness, needs, interests, or values of the person being coerced. Some think that self-protection or the prevention of harm to others is a sufficient warrant; however, as stated earlier, the mental health field lacks tools for predicting dangerousness. Others think that the individuals's own good is never a sufficient warrant for the exercise of compulsion either by the society as a whole or by its individual members.[81]

Nothing in the literature has been found that addresses the problem of maternalism and the ethical dilemmas occurring as a result of it. All nurses in all settings can interfere with a patient's liberty of action. Mental health nurses are in a particularly good position to do so, since either the patient has sought help with his behavioral problems, and this can be interpreted as giving license to staff to make decisions for his own good, or the patient has been committed by legal procedures, and this certainly can be interpreted as giving the staff the right and obligation to interfere with the patient's liberty of action.

The ideas discussed above, namely, influencing decisionmaking regarding mental status and treatment, not taking the patient seriously, and maternalism, can play a part in discussions to utilize techniques of behavior control. Nurses participate in individual and group psychotherapy, as well as in behavior modification programs. Nurses also have a great influence on decisions about drugs, such as type, dosage, and frequency. One often finds in the literature, either explicitly or implicitly, the idea that drugs make the patient more amenable to other types of therapy such as psychotherapy. Drugs also make the patient more manageable from a nursing point of view, and this raises some ethical issues around the problem of the double-agent role.

All of the ethical dilemmas raised in the preceding section involve and affect the nurse. To the extent that she is aware of them, she can examine these situations not only from a clinical perspective but also from an ethical one.

The mental health field sometimes tends to offer or promise more than it can deliver given the knowledge and technology it has available. This in itself raises ethical problems and dilemmas. The technology that is available has potential for abuse with regard to behavior control. The single most important factor in the intelligent use of such techniques is an ethically grounded clinician, who for moral reasons, hesitates in order to think through the clinical and ethical implications of his or her actions.

REFERENCES

1. London P: Personal liberty and behavior control technology. Hastings Cent Rep, February 1972, pp 4–7
2. Klerman GL: Behavior control and the limits of reform. Hastings Cent Rep, August 1975, pp 40–45
3. Goffman E: Asylums. New York, Doubleday, 1961
4. Grob GN: Mental Institutions in America: Social Policy to 1875. New York, Free Press, 1973
5. Rothman DJ: The Discovery of the Asylum: Social Order and Disorder in the New Republic. Boston, Little, Brown, 1971
6. Klerman: op cit
7. Stanton AH, Schwartz MS: The Mental Hospital. New York, Basic 1954
8. Greenblatt M, Levinson DJ, Williams R: The Patient and the Mental Hospital. Glencoe, Ill, Free Press, 1957
9. Caudill WA: A Psychiatric Hospital as a Small Society. Cambridge, Harvard University Press, 1958

10. Greenblatt M, Levinson DJ, Klerman GL: Mental Patients in Transition. Springfield, Ill, Thomas, 1961
11. Jones M: The Therapeutic Community. New York, Basic, 1953
12. ——: Beyond the Therapeutic Community. New Haven, Yale University Press, 1968
13. Szasz TS: The Myth of Mental Illness. New York, Harper & Row, 1974
14. Boyers R, Orrill R: R.D. Laing and Anti-Psychiatry. New York, Harper & Row, 1971
15. London P: Behavior Control. New York, Harper & Row, 1970
16. Orwell G: 1984. New York, Harcourt, Brace, 1959
17. Condon R: The Manchurian Candidate. New York, McGraw-Hill, 1959
18. Huxley A: Brave New World. New York, Harper & Row, 1932
19. Koestler A: Darkness at Noon. New York, Bantam, 1970
20. Halleck SL: Legal and ethical aspects of behavior control. Am J Psychiatr, April 1974, pp 381–85
21. Szasz TS: Psychiatric Justice. New York, Macmillan, 1965
22. Halleck SL: The Politics of Therapy. New York, Science House, 1971
23. Kittrie NN: The Right To Be Different. Baltimore, Johns Hopkins University Press, 1971
24. Ennis B: Prisoners of Psychiatry: Mental Patients, Psychiatry, and the Law. New York, Harcourt, Brace, Jovanovich, 1972
25. Kittrie: op cit, pp 2–4
26. Becker HS: Outsiders: Studies in the Sociology of Deviance. New York, Free Press, 1963
27. Nunnaly JC: Popular Conceptions of Mental Health. New York, Holt, Rinehart and Winston, 1961
28. Position statement on the question of adequacy of treatment. Am J Psychiatr, May 1967, pp 1458–60
29. Gulevich B, Bourne PG: Mental illness and violence. In Daniels DN, Gilula MF, Ochberg FM: Violence and the Struggle for Existence. Boston, Little, Brown, 1970, p 390
30. Rubin B: Prediction of dangerousness in mentally ill criminals. Arch Gen Psychiatr, September 1972, pp 397–407
31. Rappeport J: The Clinical Evaluation of the Dangerousness of the Mentally Ill. Springfield, Ill, Thomas, 1967
32. Halleck SC: Psychiatry and the Dilemmas of Crime. Berkeley, University of California Press, 1971
33. Stürup GK: Will this man be dangerous? In de Reuck AVS, Porter R (eds): The Mentally Abnormal Offender. Boston, Little, Brown, 1968
34. Geis T, Monahan P: The social ecology of violence. In Lickona T (eds): Moral Development and Behavior, New York, Holt, Rinehart and Winston, 1976
35. Stone AA: Mental Health and Law: A System in Transition. Rockville, Maryland, National Institute of Mental Health, 1975, p 34
36. Gaylin W: On the border of persuasion: a psychoanalytic look at coercion. Psychiatry, February 1974, pp 1–9

37. Redlich F, Mollica RF: Overview: ethical issues in contemporary psychiatry. Am J Psychiatr, February 1976, pp 125-36

38. London P: The future of psychotherapy. Hastings Cent Rep, December 1973, pp 10-13

39. Blatte H: Evaluating psychotherapies. Hastings Cent Rep, September 1973, pp 4-6

40. Ervin F: Biological intervention technologies and social control. Am Behav Sci, May-June 1975, pp 617-35

41. Burgess A: Clockwork Orange. New York, Norton, 1963

42. Augenstein L: Come Let Us Play God. New York, Harper & Row, 1969

43. Atthowe JM: Behavior modification, behavior therapy and environmental design. Am Behav Sci, May-June 1975, pp 637-56

44. Luborsky L: The latest word on comparative studies. Paper read at Society for Psychotherapy Research meeting, Denver, 1974

45. Anthony WA et al: Efficacy of psychiatric rehabilitation. Psychiatr Bull, Spring 1976 pp 44-5

46. Cowen EL: Social and community intervention. In Mussen PH, Rosenzweig MR: Annu Rev Psychol 1973

47. Holden C: Nader on mental health centers: a movement that got bogged down. Science, 177:413-15, 1972

48. Szasz TS: Problems facing psychiatry: the psychiatrist as party to conflict. In Torrey EF: Ethical Issues in Medicine. Boston, Little, Brown, 1968

49. Skinner BF: Walden Two. New York, Macmillan, 1948

50. ——: Science and Human Behavior. New York, Macmillan, 1953

51. Rogers CR: Persons or science: a philosophical question. Am Psychol 10:267-78, 1955

52. ——: Implications of recent advances in prediction and behavior control. Teachers Coll Bull 57:316-22, 1956

53. ——, Skinner BF: Some issues concerning the control of human behavior. Science, 124:1057-66, 1956

54. Jourard S: I-thou relationship versus manipulation in counseling and psychotherapy. J Individ Psychol, 15:174-79, 1959

55. ——: On the problem of reinforcement by the psychotherapist of healthy behavior in the patient. In Shaw FJ (ed): Behavioristic Approaches to Counseling and Psychotherapy. University, Alabama, University of Alabama Press, 1961

56. Krasner L: Behavior control and social responsibility. Am Psychologist 17:199-204, 1964

57. Mark VH, Ervin FR: Violence and the Brain. New York, Harper & Row, 1970

58. Psychosurgery, editorial. Lancet, July 1972, pp 69-70

59. Ballantine HT, Salter A: Psychosurgery vs. political psychiatry. Med Opinion, July 1972, pp 46-54

60. Breggin PR: The return of lobotomy and psychotherapy. Congressional Record 118, February 24, 1972, pp E1603-E1612

61. —— : Psychosurgery for the control of violence. Congressional Record 118, March 30, 1972, pp E3380–E3386
62. Miller H: Psychosurgery and Dr. Breggin. New Scientist, July 27, 1972, pp 180–90
63. Wexter DB: Violence and the brain. Harvard Law Review, 85:1489–98, 1972
64. Physical manipulation of the brain. Hastings Cent Rep, Special Suppl, May 1973, p 2
65. Mark VH, Neville R: Brain surgery in aggressive epileptics: social and ethical implications. JAMA, November 12, 1973, pp 765–72
66. Kesey K: One Flew Over the Cuckoo's Nest. New York, Viking, 1962
67. Evans W, Kline NS: Psychotropic Drugs in the Year 2000: Use by Normal Humans. Springfield, Ill, Thomas, 1971
68. Parry HJ et al: National patterns of psychotherapeutic drug use. Arch Gen Psychiatr, June 1973, pp 769–783
69. Bernstein A, Lennard HL: The American way of drugging: drugs, doctors, and junkies. Transaction/Society, May–June 1973, pp 14–25
70. Silverman M, Lee PR: Pills, Profits and Politics. Berkeley, University of California Press, 1974
71. Klerman GL: Psychotropic hedonism vs. pharmacological Calvinism. Hastings Cent Rep, September 1972, pp 1–3
72. Klerman GL: Psychotropic drugs as therapeutic agents. Hastings Cent Rep, January 1974, pp 81–93
73. Steinfels P: Confronting the other drug problem. Hastings Cent Rep, November 1972, pp 4–6
74. Veatch RM: Drugs and competing drug ethics. Hastings Cent Rep, January 1974, p 69
75. Halleck: op cit, 1974
76. Neville RC: Zalmoxis or the morals of ESB and psychosurgery. In Gaylin W: Operating on the Mind. New York, Basic, 1976
77. Bedau HA: Physical intervention to alter behavior in a primitive environment. Am Behav Sci May–June 1975, pp 657–78
78. Kittrie: op cit, pp 400–408
79. Broverman IK et al: Sex role stereotypes in clinical judgments of mental health. J Consult Clin Psychol 34:1–7, 1970
80. Rosenhan DL: On being sane in insane places. Science, January 19, 1973, pp 250–58
81. Dworkin G: Paternalism. In Gorovitz S: Moral Problems in Medicine. Englewood Cliffs, NJ, Prentice-Hall, 1976, pp 185–203

9

MENTAL RETARDATION

INTRODUCTION

The concept of developmental disability recognizes mental retardation, regardless of cause, as a facet within a spectrum of possible abnormalities.[1] The Congress enacted Public Law 91-517 in 1970 defining developmental disability as:

> ... a disability attributable to mental retardation, cerebral palsy, epilepsy or another neurological condition of an individual found by the Secretary to be closely related to mental retardation or to require treatment similar to that required for mentally retarded individuals, which disability originates before such individual attains age eighteen, which has continued or can be expect to continue indefinately, and which constitutes a substantial handicap to such individual.

Not as specific as it might be, this definition, however, does recognize disorders of adjustment, communication, locomotion, and intellectual function, and emphasizes the generally nonprogressive nature and irreversibility of these disabilities.

The Developmentally Disabled Assistance and Bill of Rights Act, Public Law 94-103, which became law in October of 1975, broadened the definition of developmental problems and the strategies for strengthening services and safeguarding individual rights. This act authorized grants for the purpose of developing services and training personnel and established a National Advisory Council on Services and Facilities for the Developmentally Disabled. The American Association on Mental Deficiency states that the term "mental retardation" refers to significantly subaverage general intellectual functioning existing concurrently with deficits in adaptive behavior and manifested during the developmental period.

Mental retardation, ultimately a social attribute, comprises at least three components: organic, functional, and social. The organic component we refer to as impairment, the functional component as disability, and the social component as handicap. Epidemiologic understanding of any disorder will differ depending on which of the three components is counted. In mild mental retardation, the rule is the absence of recognized impairment, but the presence of functional disability measured in terms of an I.Q. below a given point. The extent of social handicap varies by age and social setting.

Unfortunately, occasionally the social role of mental handicap has been conferred on a person with neither brain impairment nor functional disability. In this country and in England there have been reported cases of individuals with I.Q.'s within the normal range being placed in institutions for the retarded and so acquiring the social role of mental retardation.[2] A few seasons back a television drama, Larry, based on a true story, dealt with this problem.

Incidence measures the frequency with which disorders arise anew in a population during a specific period of time. Incidence rates in mental retardation must often obtain their data from cases clinically identified on entry to health services and, therefore, we have only approximations for two reasons. In these situations, entry into the health services for the mentally retarded rarely coincides with the onset of the disorder. Furthermore, all who have the disorder may not be represented in the sample since all mentally retarded people may not be health service consumers. Prevalence describes a disorder existing in a population at one particular time. It ignores the time of disorder onset and especially in chronic disorders it limits the inferences connecting cause and effect. Incidence gives the best view of the circumstances in which disorders arise over a period of time in a population, but depends on usage of services. Prevalence gives a good view of the needs of a specific population like the mentally retarded at a given time and is also less dependent on service usage.[3]

Although prevalence rates of mental retardation have been confounded both by definition variations of mental retardation and by the differing assessments of coexisting impairment in an individual, it has been approximated that in the United States, three percent of the general population, or 6.1 million people, have I.Q.'s of less than 70. Each year between 100,000 to 200,000 of the babies born join this group. Of the total, about 2.4 million are children and minors under 21 years of age. About 2.1 million of these children could be classified as mildly retarded, 144,000 as moderately retarded, and 120,000 as severely retarded.[4] In this country, admission records from large medical centers for children show that 25 to 30 percent of all these admissions have been for genetic disease, mental retardation, and/or congenital malformations.[5] Experts have recently catalogued almost 2000 autosomal dominant, recessive, and sex-linked disorders, but even more exist since they omitted a large number of polygenically inherited disorders.[6] These data would support the notion that few families remain untouched by genetic disorder, the results of which can range from mild to severe retardation.

The etiologic classification of mental retardation can be divided into two overall categories, genetic and acquired. The genetic category contains such examples as Down's syndrome, a chromosomal abnormality; phenylketonuria, a disorder of amino acid metabolism; Tay-Sachs, a disorder of lipid metabolism, to mention only a few conditions. Examples of acquired mental retardation can be further categorized into (1) prenatal, when infection such as rubella, toxin effects, and placental insufficiency occur; (2) perinatal, when prematurity, anoxia, or cerebral damage occur; (3) postnatal, when brain injury, infection such as meningitis, anoxia, effects of poison, and sociocultural factors such as deprivation occur. These examples given here do not exhaust the possibilities, but serve to give some idea of the complexities of mental retardation.

From 1967 through 1974, Dr. Allen Crocker, Director of the Development Evaluation Clinic, Children's Hospital, Boston, collected data on diagnostic classifications by apparent mechanism. In a total sample of 1058 mentally retarded children, he found 34 percent due to early influences on embyronic development, 27 percent due to unknown causes, 19 percent due to environmental and social problems, 11 percent due to other pregnancy problems and perinatal morbidity, five percent due to heredity issues, and four percent due to acquired childhood diseases. The exact cause of mental retardation in many cases can be most difficult to elucidate. The difficulty becomes compounded by genetic/environment interaction, prematurity, low birth-weight, and perinatal complications. The causes of mental retardation and other developmental disabilities overlap and are inextricably related in complex ways. It has been estimated that nongenetic factors may contribute as much as one-half of the total variance in I.Q. scores.[7] A detailed presentation of the causes and prevalence of mental retardation remains beyond the scope of this chapter. The above remarks serve only to indicate the magnitude and complexities of the problem and to set the stage for a discussion of other aspects of mental retardation including the ethical dilemmas involved. If the reader wishes additional material on what might be called the more biologic dimensions, the *Mental Retardation Abstracts* will be an invaluable reference. Also, any number of books as well as papers in professional journals have been published on the topic.

HISTORICAL BACKGROUND

In the United States before 1810, the majority of the mentally ill and retarded lived in homes with their families or friends or, if without a social network, they could be found in poorhouses and jails. The era of the Industrial Revolution, which brought with it waves of immigrants and a beginning shift from a rural society to an urban one, defined deviant behavior as a product of the social, political, and economic environment of the time. Social reformers viewed this environment as chaotic, disordered, and lacking stability. The traditional social procedures and institutions were breaking down and in some cases dissolving. This situation in turn created great societal stresses and strains.[8] From Europe at about this time, news of cures for insanity and deviant behavior came, with emphasis on human care in special residential institutions. This "moral treatment" developed along with the increasing belief in the physical base of certain deviant behaviors. Within this context, individuals exhibiting these behaviors became the legitimate concern of physiology and medicine.[9] By 1860, 28 of the then 33 states had built public institutions to house and care for this segment of the population. This growth in institutional care, occurring mostly between 1830 and the 1850s, became defined as the most proper treatment method.[10]

This era, which emphasized the social origins of disease, also defined idiocy and feeblemindedness as social problems. Major reformers of the day had their ideas applied, to a large extent, because they fitted the pervading assumptions about the therapeutic effects of institutionalization. And so the transformation of these institutions from residential schools to custodial asylums had support from the society at large, as well as the professionals who ran them. One writer maintains that these professionals did not necessarily invent the concept of the "menace of the feebleminded," but they did support its propagation, benefited from it, and until the 1920s opposed alternative provisions to residential segregation.[11] Essentially, the patterns of development in the institutions for the mentally retarded paralleled those used in the treatment of other forms of dependency and deviancy.

These larger social changes also had an impact on the educational system of the country. Society increasingly called on schools to train for economic, social, and civic roles, and in assuming these functions the school became the primary defender of the social order. By the 1920s, the experts and the general public assumed that by making an educational problem out of any social problem it could be effectively treated.[12] Other changes in the educational system affecting the mentally retarded also occurred during these years. The adoption of a corporate-industrial model of educational organization—in which the administration became managers, teachers the workers, the curriculum the technology, and the students the raw material for processing,[13] combined with a rise in vocationalism that lead to a definition of equality of educational opportunity[14] and the development of intelligence testing[15]—affected the role of the school vis-à-vis the mentally retarded. These changes, occurring in the first three decades of this century, combined to provide a major impetus to the emergence of special education for the mentally handicapped.

The special education movement, although gathering support from various groups, never achieved the full public acceptance enjoyed by the earlier asylum movement.[16] A variety of reasons accounted for the lack of acceptance, one of which was parental hostility that was kept in play by the school's lack of distinguishing among the different categories of children, i.e., the mentally retarded, the behaviorally disruptive, the physically handicapped, and the truant children. In short, these special classes became the dumping grounds for children that, because it lacked ways of accommodating them, the educational system could not tolerate.[17] However, an even more central problem persisted well into the latter half of this century when special education experienced a substantial growth. The original assumption underlying the special education concept remained unquestioned. The results of this central problem can best be described by employing W.I. Thomas' famous aphorism, "If men define the situation as real, then it is real in its consequences." That is to say, with regards to the mentally retarded, once a given individual's situation becomes defined, whether accurately or inaccurately, this definition becomes "the truth," which others use as the basis for their relations with that individual. The continued emphasis on I.Q. as an irremedial constant remained intact and effectively undercut the significance of psychologic and cultural variables. This lead to what Blatt calls "a predeterministic mental set," with fatalistic overtones. Education assumed that a lack of competence in traditional school requirements could be equated with a lack of competence in other areas of social activity.[18] The phenomenon of segregation for the mentally retarded in educational settings interacted with the concern over mislabeling a child as mentally retarded when in fact he was not. However, the basic assumption that the expected benefits of categorizing and labeling children always outweighed the disadvantages went unchallenged.

THE EFFECTS OF LABELING

The range of intellectual capabilities demonstrated by individuals labeled as mentally retarded varies greatly and can be divided into five categories: borderline, I.Q. 68-85; mild, I.Q. 52-67; moderate, I.Q. 36-51; severe, I.Q. 20-35; and profound, I.Q. under 20. The enormous and complex ramifications of this labeling process and the consequences of labeling will be discussed only briefly. Begab distinguishes between classification and labeling, related but differing processes, since each has a distinctive purpose and use.[19] Classification systems, designed primarily to provide statistical data about groups of similar individuals or cases, furnish the basis for measuring incidence, prevalence, characteristics, and other information, including the success of programs established to prevent or ameliorate the condition.[20] Such a procedure as classification has many problems. The most basic problem stems from the difficulty of any effort to categorize the totality and complexity of a human being. No matter how multidimensional the classification methods, their imperfections and inadequacies will soon become apparent. An interesting paradox that compounds this serious problem in classifying any group can be noted. The more knowledge that science develops about a given entity, in this case mental retardation, the more difficult classification becomes because of the additional dimensions and complexities. The classification system presents special problems in dealing with individuals in the mild or moderate categories. Frequent discrepancies occur between adaptive behavior and measured intelligence, making it difficult to determine who should be classified in which category. These problems may be further compounded by the sociopolitical processes at play in the society at any given time. For example, in recent years, questions have been raised about the use of I.Q. testing as a basis for classifying and placing individuals in programs. The limitations of I.Q. tests and the possible errors in using them points to their disadvantage as the only source of information used to classify people. Other problems can be identified, including the presumed cultural bias controversy[21] and the difficulty in assessing social competence. The I.Q. and social competence tests must be supplemented by life history data, biomedical information, and clinical judgment.

Classification would not be possible without the labeling process. The label of mental retardation, like all such labels, serves as a shorthand way of saying a number of things about an individual or group. Although labels may be necessary to facilitate communication, they do tend to conjure up stereotypes, especially socially defined pejorative ones, of the labeled person. For example, people hold an image of the alcoholic as a skid-row bum and not as the business executive, although in this latter group alcoholism constitutes a problem of some magnitude. Labels, in and of themselves, are not inherently bad, although they can, and sometimes do, come in for abuse. With the mental retardation label, one abuse derives from overlooking the vast range of individual differences found in the people so labeled. This abuse can lead us to interact with all mentally retarded persons as if no differences existed. All of us, including the mentally retarded, gain and maintain our concept of self from interaction with others. If we constantly respond to a retarded individual in stereotyped ways, then he continually receives feedback about himself that may be based more on our preconceptions and stereotypes than on the individual himself. This could lead to a self-fulfilling prophecy, in that the mentally retarded person begins to respond to us based on our notion of him. For example, if we view him as dependent and unable to do for himself, then he may behave to fit this view of him. The labeling concept in mental retardation remains complex and the voluminous literature on the topic does not always provide us with conclusive data regarding the multiple dimensions of the process.[22-27] Although some believe this process causes great harm by stigmatizing, others point out that once labeled accurately, a mentally retarded individual has access to beneficial services. Perhaps it will help if we remember that the mental retardation label is the most stigmatizing of all in our society.[28]

ATTITUDES TOWARD THE RETARDED

One of the central concerns regarding the mental retardation label is the attitude that society holds toward this population. The social context, out of which the label comes, reflects the attitudes that also in large part determine society's reaction to the mentally retarded. Major attention has been given to the negative consequences of classifying and labeling children as mentally retarded. These studies have tended to search for evidence to illustrate the nature and manifestations of stigma, without examining possible beneficial consequences of the classification system.[29]

The rationale for research on attitudes toward the retarded, or any other deviant population, rests on the assumption that when a society has more favorable attitudes toward such a group, more enlightened treatment of them ensues. The other side of this assumption, negative attitudes that lead to the group remaining in a more unenviable societal position than necessary, has been documented. In an era such as our own, when the emphasis has shifted to keeping the retarded in the community by having them participate in community-based programs, the attitudes of and acceptance by the local residents become a crucial factor in the success or failure of such an endeavor. As part of this change, some school systems have abolished their segregated, special classes and have reintegrated the mentally retarded students into the regular school classes. The general idea of integration takes into account the student's ability to handle the situation and the existence of separate programs as needed. For example, a plan may include integration for social and nonacademic portions of the curriculum with special teaching in resource programs. This concept of integration does not imply that such programs for the mentally retarded would be to the detriment of more competent students.

The general public views the retarded as a mongoloid or a brain-damaged individual.[30] Although professionals in the field know that the overwhelming proportion of retardation can be attributed to cultural and/or environmental differences and not to organic and/or genetic abnormalities, the above view among the public persists. Patterns have emerged from numerous community attitude surveys. The public has more favorable attitudes toward the mildly mentally retarded than toward the severely retarded. They often confuse mental retardation with mental illness and show a general ignorance regarding the retarded themselves and the services available to them.[31] In addition, the neurologically disabled, e.g., cerebral palsy and aphasia, may be both mislabeled and misunderstood as mentally retarded because of their functional disabilities. Research does not consistently indicate that contact with retarded people results in more favorable attitudes toward them.[32-34]

The research on peer attitudes, relying in the main on sociometric instruments, shows the response to mildly retarded children in the school system. A number of studies demonstrate that regardless of the particular educational model employed, educable mentally retarded children are not so well accepted by their peers as are nonretarded children.[35-37] One study indicated that peer groups accepted the educable mentally retarded from a higher socioeconomic status better than they did those from a lower status.[38] Another study concluded that special or regular class placement does not affect the neighborhood interaction patterns of retarded children, since the other children ignore them regardless of placement.[39]

Little research has been conducted on the attitudes of those health professionals most likely to come into contact with the mentally retarded. Studies on the attitudes of school teachers have been undertaken that may throw some light on one aspect of the immediate future when more retarded children attend regular classrooms. Studies show that regular education teachers do not have especially positive attitudes toward children with a mental retardation label[40] and the length of teaching experience either does not promote positive changes in attitudes[41] or else results in more unfavorable attitudes.[42] Numerous studies have documented the fact that a primary function of educational institutions has become the allocation of persons to adult roles and statuses in the larger society.[43-46] The attitudes of teachers, which have been shown to have a significant effect on children's academic performance,[47] takes on special meaning within this context. The extent to which teachers' attitudes or expectations affect retarded children's performance remains open to question but it may influence his social status among his peer group if nothing else.[48]

In the past, the school nurse has encountered the less mildly retarded child in the school system. At present, the trend is toward accommodating the more severely and multiply handicapped with physical and mental disability in the public school system. Until recently these children would have been either in a day-care program or in no program at all. So the role of the school vis-à-vis this population will grow in importance. In addition, now that this trend will keep the mentally retarded out of total institutions, they will seek medical services in the general hospital as needed. Therefore, the hospital nurse will more likely have contact with this group than in the past. These changes have occurred within the newly expanded legal and civil rights for the mentally retarded.

THE LEGAL AND CIVIL RIGHTS OF THE RETARDED

The interaction between the law and mental retardation presents the most confused, ambiguous picture in the entire mental health area.[49] A clearly demonstrated example of this situation can be found in the legal standard of mental retardation that serves as the threshold label invoked in statutes authorizing confinement. In at least five states, the statutes read that mental deficiency shall mean mental deficiency as defined by appropriate Clinical Authorities.[50] The law, in these cases, totally abdicates responsibility to clinicians and this may lead to the practice of unregulated admissions and the abuse of the retarded person's civil liberties. The typical statutory definition of mental deficiency uses such phrases as "incapable of managing himself and his affairs" and "for whose own welfare or that of others, supervision, guidance, care, or control is necessary or admissible."[51] These statutes recognize that the justification of confinement in these cases can not be on the danger-to-others concept, but rather must be on the idea that it benefits the retarded person, his family, or the community. The effectiveness of these statutes is limited, since most retarded individuals become confined while still minors and therefore they have no recourse to a court of law.

Murdock identified three interacting areas affecting the civil rights of the mentally retarded: guardianship, institutionalization, and education.[52] Deeply rooted in our legal system and our general notions of society lies the belief that parents are the natural guardians of children. This belief implies a compatibility of interest between parent and child and the ability on the parent's part to care for and represent the child in his dealings with the institutions of society. However, as the President's Committee on Mental Retardation points out, the provisions in most states largely consider or assume the retarded person to be without rights, deny him due process or the equal protection of the law.[53] Moreover, a conflict of interest may exist between the parent and the child. For example, the parent may be motivated to seek institutionalization for a number of reasons other than the best interests of the child himself, i.e., perceived stigma of mental retardation, economic stress, physical and mental frustration, consideration for other children in the family. The retarded child's best interest may well lie in living with his family and in the community, but theirs may not lie in keeping him.[54] The film, *Who Should Survive*,[55] graphically illustrates a most fundamental conflict of interest in depicting the real situation where, because of the parents' decision, the hospital withheld minor corrective surgery from a Down's syndrome infant with an intestinal obstruction. The infant died a slow death from dehydration. This situation raises numerous ethical dilemmas that will be discussed in another section of this chapter.

The rights of any institutionalized person can be abused and this may be especially true for the mentally retarded. While many rights to which the retarded are entitled have been outlined, including the right to visitation by family members at all reasonable hours,[56] the right to receive compensation for their labor,[57] and the right to normal relationships with the opposite sex,[58] probably the most crucial rights for this group are the right to a humane physical and psychologic environment and the right to adequate treatment. The need for judicial recognition of constitutional standards with respect to the care of the institutionalized retarded arose from the abuses of these rights, many of which have been documented in legal testimony.

The genesis of a legally enforceable right to treatment concept appeared in a 1960 article advocating the rights of the mentally ill, but did not mention the mentally retarded.[59] The first significant judicial development occurred in 1966 when the District of Columbia court determined that the 1964 Hospitalization of the Mentally Ill Act did provide a right to treatment which could be judicially enforced.[60]

Subsequent court decisions have further defined the right to treatment and have expanded it to include a constitutional right to the "least restrictive alternative." This means that when someone becomes ill and in need of treatment, but is not dangerous to self or others, he cannot legally be confined in the most restrictive setting, such as a locked hospital ward. The rationale for this principle is that "commitment entails an extraordinary deprivation of liberty" and that "such a drastic curtailment of the rights of citizens must be narrowly, even grudgingly, constructed in order to avoid deprivation of liberty without due process of law."[61] Not until 1972, when the third decision in the *Wyatt* v. *Stickney* case mentioned the right to habilitation for the mentally retarded, did this group receive consideration. The court defined habilitation as "the process by which the staff of the institution assists the resident to acquire and maintain those life skills which enable him to cope more effectively with the demands on his own person and of his environment and to raise the level of his physical, mental, and social efficiency."[62] Habilitation, although not limited to, includes programs of formal, structured education and treatment. This extended the right to treatment in medical terms to include education. Further refinement of this concept encompassed the nature of the living conditions generally, whether each patient has an individualized plan, and generally enjoys a humane psychologic and physical environment.

Although the 1969 President's Committee on Retardation estimated that approximately 60 percent of the retarded school age children were not receiving an education,[63] Murdock maintains that the prospects for the retarded appear the highest in the area of education. He bases his statement on several factors. A federal constitutional basis for arguing that the retarded are entitled to a public education now exist. Additionally, many state constitutions require the establishment of a public educational system open to all. The requirement of upgrading the quality of habilitation in state institutions and the concomitant cost spiral resulting creates tremendous pressures to provide services to the retarded outside of the traditional, huge, warehouselike institutions.[64]

To expect the judiciary to correct all the wrongs experienced by the mentally retarded is a quixotic notion, but recent events in the legal system have opened the courtroom door to the advocates of the retarded. In this process, the American public has had an opportunity to gain insight into the dimensions, including the legal and ethical ones, involved in caring for the retarded children and adults in our society.

The United Nations General Assembly in 1971 adopted a declaration on the rights of the retarded that reads:

> Reaffirming faith in human rights and fundamental freedoms and in the principles of peace, of the dignity and worth of the human person and of social justice proclaimed in the Charter,

Recalling the principles of the Universal Declaration of Human Rights, the International Covenants on Human Rights, the Declaration of the Rights of the Child and the standards already set for social programs in the Constitutions, conventions, accommodations and resolutions of the International Labour Organization, the United Nations Educational, Scientific and Cultural Organization, the World Health Organization, the United Nations Children's Fund and of other organizations concerned,

Emphasizing that the Declaration on Social Progress and Development has proclaimed the necessity of protecting the rights and assuring the welfare and rehabilitation of the physically and mentally disadvantaged,

Bearing in mind the necessity of assisting mentally retarded persons to develop their abilities in various fields of activities and of promoting their integration as far as possible in normal life,

Aware that certain countries, at their present stage of development, can devote only limited efforts to this end,

Proclaims this Declaration on the Rights of Mentally Retarded Persons and calls for national and international action to ensure that it will be used as a common basis and frame of reference for the protection of these rights:

1. The mentally retarded person has, to the maximum degree of feasibility, the same rights as other human beings.
2. The mentally retarded person has a right to proper medical care and physical therapy and to such education, training, rehabilitation and guidance as will enable him to develop his ability and maximum potential.
3. The mentally retarded person has a right to economic security and to a decent standard of living. He has a right to perform productive work or to engage in any other meaningful occupation to the fullest possible extent of his capabilities.
4. Whenever possible, the mentally retarded person should live with his own family or with foster parents and participate in different forms of community life. The family with which he lives should receive assistance. If care in an institution becomes necessary, it should be provided in surroundings and other circumstances as close as possible to those of normal life.
5. The mentally retarded person has a right to a qualified guardian when this is required to protect his personal well-being and interests.
6. The mentally retarded person has a right to protection from exploitation, abuse and degrading treatment. If prosecuted for any offense, he shall have a right to due process of law with full recognition being given to his degree of mental responsibility.

7. Whenever mentally retarded persons are unable because of the severity of their handicap to exercise all their rights in a meaningful way, or it should become necessary to restrict or deny some or all of these rights, the procedure used for that restriction or denial of rights must contain proper legal safeguards against every form of abuse. This procedure must be based on an evaluation of the social capability of the mentally retarded person by qualified experts and must be subject to periodic review and to the rights of appeal to higher authorities.

More recently, a New York Times article reported that the number of handicapped people with diverse disabilities, such as physical handicaps, blindness, and mental retardation, taken together total to approximately 50 million people. Arbitrary exclusion from society has produced an aggressive civil rights movement focused on the right to mobility, education, and jobs. Thousands of disabled persons were reported picketing, filing suits, and lobbying for the equal protection promised, but not received, under the Fourteenth Amendment. Militant groups such as Disabled for Action and the National Federation for the Blind accuse traditional service groups like the March of Dimes, Easter Seals, and the American Foundation for the Blind of encouraging paternalism and insensitivity toward the handicapped.[65]

GENETIC SCREENING

Governments have special concerns for the health of citizens. For example, many nations have statutory programs to provide for the control of contagious diseases. There have also been times when the state legally forced a person to have treatment even when no discernible risk to society from the illness could be demonstrated. The boundaries of permissible government activities to regulate more generally the health of society as a whole have been delineated, in past, by constitutional constraints such as: the guarantee of the freedom to religious convictions; the guarantee that no person be deprived of life, liberty, or property without due process of the law; and the guarantee that no state shall deny to any person within its jurisdiction the equal protection of the law. The doctrine of Fundamental Interests holds that certain human activities not mentioned in the Bill of Rights deserve special judicial protection. One of these activities, privacy or the right to be left alone, has slowly expanded to include rights of personal decision making.[66] No absolute and clear delineation of the outer limits of government action pursuant to the public health power can be made. The state's power to order an individual to undergo a medical procedure, such as immunization, sterilization, blood tests, and x-rays, has far-reaching implications. The potential of this power for both evil and good is obvious and any proposal for the extension of the power deserves very careful scrutiny.[67] Genetic-screening legislation represents one such extension of this power.

Genetic-screening legislation, written to provide for the detection of both treatable disease and carrier status, received little public discussion prior to passage. Between 1962 and 1971, 43 states and the District of Columbia passed laws mandating neonatal screening for phenylketonuria, referred to as PKU.[68] By 1972, 12 states and the District of Columbia had legislated sickle cell anemia screening laws.[69] This legislation, written to influence childbearing decisions by heterozygous couples and thereby reduce the number of births of affected children, overlooked the dangers implicit in such laws. Because of the association of sickle cell anemia with only one race, screening laws confronted an unusual equal protection problem. This situation became further compounded by the fact that these laws failed to provide for confidentiality of test information, availability of competent, free genetic-counseling services, and programs to educate the general public about genetic disease. Similar problems, encountered in other disease-specific legislation, such as laws regarding Tay-Sachs disease and Cooley's anemia, raise larger questions as to the appropriateness and effectiveness of this multiplication of disease-specific laws.[70]

Genetic-screening programs have the goals of treatment and reduction of the number of births of affected persons. The major traditional goal has been treatment of identified persons with a given condition; however, the other goal has increasingly received attention within the context of developing health care priorities and allocating resources. This raises a myriad of ethical issues.

At present, the government seems to favor the "pure voluntarism" model in the area of eugenic legislation. Screening legislation should be written with a clear understanding of the immediate potential risks and benefits and a recognition of policy implications. In addition, these laws should safeguard the integrity of the individual who will be tested. It is true that mandatory screening laws would possibly achieve a more rapid reduction of genetic disease than would voluntary legislation; however, the unique potential that genetic data holds for subtle social and political discrimination can be viewed as a risk which outweighs the envisioned benefit.[71]

GENETIC COUNSELING

For Milunsky, the premise that human rights of personal inviolability include the fundamental right to life with a self-determined destiny and the right to marry and procreate served to establish the guiding principles in genetic counseling.[72] These rights delineate the providence of moral autonomy and individual privacy in decisions about procreation.

The World Health Organization Expert Committee on genetic counseling has endorsed the nondirective approach with parents.[73] Although this practice has been recommended, Sorenson's research points to the difficulties confronting counselors when the evidence shows that 54 percent of counselors tend to leave all decisions to parents, while 64 percent of this same group reported that they informed parents in a way that would guide them toward an "appropriate" decision.[74] The intrinsic danger involved in this paradox found in nondirective counseling, as well as in the more direct counseling approach, is the possible insinuation by the counselor of his or her own religious, racial, eugenic, or other dictates into the counseling encounter.

Capron argues that parents have a legal right to receive full information including options, risks, benefits, and consequences available or foreseeable as they deliberate their decision about procreation.[75] This takes on special relevance with the changes in the timing of counseling. Parents, in the past, usually received genetic counseling after the birth of a child with genetic disease. Recent advances in genetic technology, such as prenatal diagnosis and carrier detection, enable parents at risk to receive counseling prior to having children.

Another type of counseling, which might be called Family Adjustment counseling, becomes an important service in those families who have a newborn developmentally defective infant. Some of the same counseling difficulties, paradoxes, and ethical dilemmas can be encountered here as well as in genetic counseling.

ETHICAL DILEMMAS

Any discussion of ethical dilemmas and the mentally retarded must take into account the concept of respect for persons. Private morality concerns itself with respecting the distinctive human endowment as we find it in ourselves, whereas public morality is concerned with respecting the distinctive human endowment as we find it in others. Private and public morality therefore represent two aspects of a single, fundamental moral principle.[76] We feel brotherly love, agape, respect toward those regarded as persons. This notion leaves open the possibility of debate as to who or what properly and truly constitutes a person we are to regard with respect. Traditionally, it has been assumed that basic to the distinctive endowment of a human being is his ability to reason. Kant, a typical and supreme representative of the Age of Enlightenment, developed the thesis that possession of a rational will was the quality that gives a person absolute worth.[77] So for Kant and the others influenced by him, this became the quality of the generic self or the distinctive endowment of human beings that made a human a person to be respected for no other reason than that he was a human person. The philosophical arguments that have surrounded the Kantian thesis may not be known to many people; nevertheless, this thinking has influenced, directly or indirectly, our attitudes toward a number of groups including the mentally retarded.

The concept "person" is already an evaluative concept with something of the force of "that which makes a human being valuable" implied in it. But the questions remain, Why do we respect or value a person? What makes a human being a person?[78] In the field of developmental disability, as we move along the continuum from borderline retarded to profoundly retarded, do we perceive each individual as a person or do we draw the line based on moral reasoning, and think only of some on the continuum as persons whom we respect? The consequences of society's definition of person and where we draw the line around that category have crucial relevance for the mentally retarded as well as for society as a whole.

In addition, as scientific advances make the genetic control of man a real possibility, the alterations of the human race have been taken out of the realm of science fiction and put into the hands of laboratory scientists. Profound ethical and anthropologic issues are raised by the possible future technical, biologic control and change of the human species. The fascinating prospects of man's limitless self-modification make even more urgent the need to articulate the possible line of moral reasoning concerning them.[79] In 1969, the Rand Corporation developed a table of human expectations that included: artificial inovulation by 1995; routine animal cloning by 2005; widespread human cloning by 2020; routine breeding of hybrids and specialized human mutants by the year 2025.[80] Discussions of the moral questions raised by the new biology have already begun. Importantly, these discussions as reported by the press have included public debate in such places as Massachusetts and California. Basically, the ethical dilemmas in genetic control are so fundamental to our traditional definition of personhood that the moral reasoning used to explore the possible solutions to these dilemmas for future generations must include the profound, basic fact that a true society is sustained by the sense of human dignity.[81]

Lappé points out that the development of a eugenic policy, aimed at improving the genetic quality of whole populations over time, raises many questions of value. For example, from a genetic perspective, what constitutes a "good" demographic profile for a nation? Would any attempt to attain such a profile conflict with the values and needs of the populace? What human characteristics should such a policy favor? What constitutes a deleterious gene for an individual, family, ethnic group, or an entire population?[82]

One presently functioning procedure in genetic control that we more and more take for granted, genetic screening, also presents ethical dilemmas. Ought the government require every potential parent to undergo screening for possible genetic disease? If so, how will the data indicating genetic problems be used, by whom, and for what purposes? Does obtaining and using such data infringe on the rights of the individuals who have been screened? What are the risks and benefits involved in this information for the couple and for society? Once a couple knows that they may produce a developmentally handicapped child, what obligations, if any, do they have to each other, any other members of their family, and to society as a whole? Do they have an inalienable right to knowingly produce a disabled child? Do they have an obligation not to have children? Who will determine their rights and obligations, on what basis, and what will be the consequences of such determination?

Once a developmentally compromised child is born, then another set of ethical questions arises. Guttman, in discussing how to proceed when dealing with a child who has multiple congenital anomalies, makes the point that withholding treatment may favor the development of active euthanasia, hitherto avoided by health professionals and condemned by all religions. The ethical dilemmas involved in active and passive euthanasia, raising the question as to whether letting die is the same as killing, have been discussed at length in Chapter 7 on dying and death. Guttman developed a classification system for these infants. Category one includes infants with abnormalities incompatible with life if untreated, but in whom total recovery can be expected after surgical management. Category two includes infants with severe anomalies incompatible with life and not correctable. Category three includes infants with correctable abnormalities that would be lethal if untreated, but who would be permanently abnormal even if treated with surgery. And finally, category four includes infants with abnormalities that could possibly be fatal, and in whom corrective surgery would result in a more severe handicap.[83] Obviously, categories three and four create serious ethical problems. One consideration in the moral reasoning here may become the issue of the quality of life. Some would hold that the issue is not the prospective quality of life to be preserved, but that of the most basic right enjoyed by every person, the right of life itself. Frequently, the option for a life of quality becomes linked to economic indicators and the issue of resources and distributive justice.[84] Some would argue for the right to life for all persons regardless of its quality. Others would either not define the profoundly retarded as persons with a right to life or would argue that the risks and benefits for the retarded must be weighed against the duties and obligations which society has for all its members.

If moral reasoning favors the mentally retarded, then the obligations and duties of society to safeguard their basic rights become the focus of concern. Crocker and Cushna outline those "normal rights" of this group that must be defended or sought to include the right to: family living, educational opportunities, treatment and habilitation services, employment, support in the development of contracts, and confidentiality in personal records. They also outline "special rights" to include qualified advocacy and guardianship capacity, protection against use of drugs and behavior modification techniques, including experimental procedures, counseling and safeguards regarding reproduction, and intelligent exposure to life situations involving risk.[85]

In response to the outcry over the sterilization in 1973 of two young black women, the federal government imposed a moratorium on utilizing federal funds to sterilize anyone under 21 years of age or the mentally incompetent. One aspect of the sterilization argument is the parameters of governmental control. No one, critic or advocate of regulations, believes that anyone should ever be coerced into accepting sterilization. Advocates of regulation believe that abuses occur frequently enough, especially with vulnerable groups such as minors, the poor, and the mentally incompetent, to warrant strong controls. Critics of such regulations do not believe such abuse is the case and maintain that some, including the poor and the mentally incompetent, have actually been abused by being denied sterilization based on the arbitrary judgments of a physician or hospital. This moral dilemma raises the question as to whether any of the mentally retarded should be sterilized and if so, which ones, on what grounds, and on whose consent shall it be done. Some believe that sterilization ought to be available for people who are sexually active but unable to care for a child. Others believe that only the mentally retarded capable of giving informed consent should ever be candidates for sterilization.[86,87]

Since the ethical dilemmas of informed consent in research have been discussed elsewhere, the problem of mentally retarded individuals participating in research studies will be mentioned only briefly here. As indicated, certain groups, such as the mentally ill, children, prisoners, and the mentally retarded, present special ethical problems as research subjects because of the informed consent requirement and the possibility of coercion. One study, the Willowbrook experiments,[88] conducted on mentally retarded institutionalized children, raised numerous ethical questions and led to a debate about obtaining informed consent and from whom, the relationship between the consenting parent and the institutionalized child, the ethics of undertaking research on such a group when it is neither therapeutic nor likely to benefit the patients in any way but can only be classified as an experimental procedure that may or may not benefit other people in the future.[89-92]

In summary, the ethical dilemmas discussed with regard to the mentally retarded can be listed as: concept of person, how we define it and the consequences the definition has; genetic control and eugenic policy as they affect the individual, the family, an ethnic group, a nation, the world, and future generations; the role of genetic screening and counseling; problems encountered by the mentally retarded in institutions and in the community regarding their rights, and the moral reasoning that society uses in balancing its resources and values to determine the risks and benefits for the individual and for society itself.

ETHICAL IMPLICATIONS FOR NURSING PRACTICE

With some few exceptions, recent journal articles focused on nursing practice and mental retardation have dealt with ethical dilemmas either indirectly or by implication or not at all.[92-100] Perhaps this lack reflects, among other things, the profound nature of these ethical dilemmas and the difficulties we experience in coming to grips with the emotions that the mentally retarded elicit in us. When we encounter a physically handicapped person we can experience the encounter as an affront to our own personal integrity in that we realize the fragility of the world that we take for granted. The old adage, "There but for the grace of God, go I," implies a universal vulnerability in a world over which we do not have absolute control. An encounter with the mentally retarded can be experienced as an affront to the most fundamental core of our own personhood. We react to this affront with a variety of feelings, including thankfulness that we are as we are and guilt that we live in a world of "haves" and "have nots." Another adage comes to mind, "I complained because I had no shoes until I saw the man who had no feet." Old adages have much collected folk wisdom in them and tell us some things about ourselves.

In attempting to cope with such an encounter, commonly experienced feelings of repulsion and disgust can not only prevent us from examining the roots of our reaction, they can also have wide-ranging effects on our definition of the situation and on how, or if we deal with the moral claims that the mentally retarded have on us as an individual. Our attitudes also will determine how we think the resources of society should be allocated and how much of what we think the mentally retarded should receive. The concept, distributive justice, provides us with a moral framework within which to make these decisions.

Obviously, the nurse must first sort out her own feelings about and attitudes toward the mentally retarded. Such a sorting out will need to take into account the concept of personhood and where she draws the line, if at all, with regard to the extent of the retardation and the consequences of such action. Such questions raised will be: What attitudes do I have toward the mentally retarded? What attitudes should I have and why? Do I tend to stereotype all the mentally retarded and view them as a category rather than as individuals with differences? What moral principles have I used to think through my ethical position vis-à-vis the retarded? What moral claims do the retarded have on me as a professional? What moral claims do they have on society? How do we articulate these claims within the concept of distributive justice?

Parents have reported less than helpful reactions from others ranging from too much sympathy to denial of any sort of problem, to rejection.[101] These and other reactions grounded in negative attitudes toward the mentally retarded can hinder the nurse from performing the basic functions of her role to say nothing of the quality of her caring. It can only be assumed that the nurses working directly with the retarded and their families over a period of time have developed a moral position that enables them to provide all of the care required in the situation, while at the same time protecting the rights of these patients. Medicine has been accused of paternalism, but nursing needs to examine its activities especially with such patients as the mentally retarded and the mentally ill, to ascertain the extent of the maternalism that we inflict on others. In the sense in which any of us can ever be said to be at home in the world, we are at home not through dominating but through caring for the other in ways that permit both to grow.

More problems may occur for the school nurse, the community nurse, or the nurse in the acute-care setting, whose encounters with the retarded have been less often and of less intensity. In dealing with the ethical dilemmas of mental retardation, one focus that may be helpful, and which, as indicated, has received much attention, is the rights of the retarded person. The official statement of the American Association on Mental Deficiency makes the point that in all activities, designing facilities and organizing services, allocating funds and other resources, participating in the legislative or judicial process, teaching, conducting research, and "most of all, when participating directly in the treatment, training, and habilitation of retarded persons," the rights of these individuals should serve as the foundation of all else.

For the nurse in the neonatal intensive care unit, the possible dilemma that she faces around the issue of letting the infant die because he is retarded will call for moral reasoning with regard to the part she can or can not play in this drama. It can only be hoped that the environment in such a unit will encourage open discussion of these ethical dilemmas in all their complex points.

As the field of genetics further advances, nurses, both practitioners and educators, individually and collectively, along with other health professionals and concerned citizens, must become more knowledgeable about the implications of this research. Decisions and research findings in this field affect all of us living now as well as future generations. The need to weigh the potential risks and possible benefits on the future course of human evolution has been addressed often recently. Our deep-rooted concepts of ourselves and our relationship to the universe will be reappraised in this process. This has enormous consequences, not only for the mentally retarded but for all of us. Value judgments inevitably will play an important part in determining the direction society takes on this scientific and ethical issue. One can only wonder if the insights and humility gained from encounters with the mentally retarded will help in this awesome task before us.[102,103] As the largest segment of the health industry, nurses should have some valuable input into this debate. In all of these ethical dilemmas, the moral principles of justice and utility, or the greatest possible balance of good over evil, have a part in our concept of obligations to the mentally retarded, as well as to the rest of us, now and in the future.

REFERENCES

1. Milunsky A: Introduction. In Milunsky A: The Prevention of Genetic Diseases and Mental Retardation. Philadelphia, Sunders, 1975, p 3
2. Stein Z, Susser M: Public health and mental retardation. In Begab MJ, Richardson SA: The Mentally Retarded and Society. Baltimore, University Park Press, 1974, p 64
3. Ibid., p 54
4. National Association for Retarded Children, Facts on Mental Retardation 5, Washington, DC, 1971
5. Clow CL, Fraser FC, Laberge C, et al: On the application of knowledge to the patient with genetic disease. In Steinberg AG, Bearn AG: Progress in Medical Genetics, vol 9, New York, Grune & Stratton, 1973, p 159
6. McKusick VA: Mendelian Inheritance in Man. Baltimore, Johns Hopkins Press, 1971
7. Motulsky AG: Population genetics of mental retardation. In Jervis GA: Expanding Concepts in Mental Retardation. Springfield, Ill, Thomas, 1968, p 13
8. Rothman DJ: The Discovery of the Asylum: Social Order and Disorder in the New Republic. Boston, Little, Brown, 1971
9. Dain N: Concepts of Insanity in the United States, 1789–1865. New Brunswick, NJ, Rutgers University Press, 1964
10. Lazerson M: Educational institutions and mental subnormality: notes on writing a history. In Begab MJ, Richardson SA: op cit, p 37
11. Wolfensberger W: The origin and nature of our institutional models. In Kugel RB, Wolfensberger W: Changing Patterns in Residential Services for the Mentally Retarded. Washington, DC, President's Committee on Mental Retardation, 1969, pp 59–171
12. Cremin LA: The Transformation of the School. New York, Knopf, 1962
13. Spring J: Education and the Rise of the Corporate State. Boston, Beacon, 1972
14. Lazerson M, Grubb WN: American Education and Vocationalism, 1870–1970. New York, Teachers College Press, 1974

15. Haller M: Eugenics: Hereditarian Attitudes in American Thought. New Brunswick, NJ, Rutgers University Press, 1963
16. Lazerson M: In Begab MJ, Richardson SA: op cit, p 49
17. White House Conference on Child Health and Protection: Special Education. New York, Century, 1931
18. Blatt B: Some persistently recurring assumptions concerning the mentally subnormal. In Rothstein JH: Mental Retardation. New York, Holt, Rinehart, and Winston, 1961, pp 113–25
19. Begab MJ: Trends and issues. In Begab MJ, Richardson SA: op cit, pp 26–29
20. Grossman H: Manual on Terminology and Classification in Mental Retardation. Washington, American Association for Mental Deficiency, 1973
21. Anastasi A: Psychological Testing. New York, Macmillan, 1968
22. Edgerton RB: The Cloak of Competence—Stigma in the Lives of the Mentally Retarded. Berkeley, University of California Press, 1967
23. Goffman I: Stigma—Notes on the Management of Spoiled Identity. Englewood Cliffs, NJ, Prentice-Hall, 1963
24. Kleck R, Ono H, Hastorf AH: The effects of physical deviance upon face-to-face interaction. Human Relations 19:425–36, 1966
25. Lippman L: Attitudes Toward the Handicapped. Springfield, Ill, Thomas, 1972
26. MacMillan DA, Jones RL, Aloia GF: The mentally retarded label: a theoretical analysis and review of research. Am J Ment Defic 79:241–61, 1974
27. Mercer JR: Labeling the Mentally Retarded. Berkeley, University of California Press, 1973
28. Edgerton RB, Sabagh G: From mortification to aggrandizement: changing self-concepts in the careers of the mentally retarded. Psychiatry 25:263–72, 1962
29. Richardson SA: Reaction to mental subnormality. In Begab MJ, Richardson SA: op cit, p 95
30. Gottwald H: Public awareness about mental retardation. Research Monograph, Arlington, Va, Council for Exceptional Children, 1970
31. Gottlieb J: Public, peer, and professional attitudes. In Begab MJ, Richardson SA: op cit, p 102
32. Phelps WR: Attitudes related to the employment of mentally retarded. Am J Ment Defic 69:575–85, 1965
33. Hollinger CS, Jones RL: Community attitudes toward slow learners and mental retardates. Ment Retard 8:19–23, 1970
34. Gottlieb J, Corman L: Public attitudes toward mentally retarded children. Am J Ment Defic 80:72–80, 1975
35. Johnson GO: Social position of mentally handicapped children in regular grades. Am J Ment Defic 55:60–89, 1950
36. Gottlieb J, Davis JE: Social acceptance of EMRS during overt behavioral interaction. Am J Ment Defic 78:141–43, 1973
37. Iano RP, Ayers D, Heller AB, McGettingan, Walker VS: Sociometric

status of retarded children in an integrative program. Except Child 40: 267–71, 1974

38. Monroe JD, Howe CE: Effects of integration and social class on the acceptance of retarded adolescents. Educ Train Ment Retard 6:20–24, 1971

39. Meyerowitz JH: Self-derogations in young retardates and special class placement. Ment Retard 5:23–26, 1967

40. Combs RH, Harper JL: Effects of labels on attitudes of educators toward handicapped children. Except Child 33:399–403, 1967

41. Alper S, Retish PM: A comparative study of the effects of student teaching in the attitudes of students in special education, elementary education, and secondary education. Train School Bull 69:70–77, 1972

42. Shotel JR, Iano RP, McGettigan JF: Teacher attitude associated with the integration of handicapped children. Except Child 38:677–83, 1972

43. Parsons T: The school class as a social system. Harvard Ed Rev 29:297–315, 1959

44. Turner R: Sponsored and contest mobility and the school system. Am Soc Rev 25:855–67, 1960

45. Cicourel A, Kitsuse J: The Educational Decisionmakers. New York, Bobbs-Merrill, 1963

46. Jencks C et al: Inequality: A Reassessment of the Effect of Family and Schooling in America. New York, Basic, 1972

47. Rosenthal R, Jacobson L: Pygmalion in the Classroom: Teacher Expectation and Pupil's Intellectual Development. New York, Holt, Rinehart, and Winston, 1968

48. Lapp ER: A study of the social adjustment of slow-learning children who were assigned part-time to regular classes. Am J Ment Defic 62:254–62, 1959

49. Stone AA: Mental Health and Law: A System in Transition, Washington, Dept. of HEW, National Institute of Mental Health, 1975, pp 119–40

50. Brakel S, Rock R: The Mentally Disabled and the Law. Chicago, University of Chicago Press, 1971, pp 98–102

51. Ennis B, Friedman PR: Legal Rights of the Mentally Handicapped. New York, Practising Law Institute, 1973, pp 15–101

52. Murdock CW: Civil rights of the mentally retarded: some critical issues. Notre Dame Lawyer, October 1972, pp 133–88

53. The President's Committee on Mental Retardation, The Decisive Decade, Washington, DC, 1970

54. Wyatt v Stickney 325F Supp 781 M.D. Ala., 1971

55. Who Should Survive? Washington, DC, Joseph P. Kennedy, Jr. Foundation, 1971

56. Brakel S, Rock R: op cit

57. Townsend v Treadway, Civil No. 6500, M.D. Tenn., 1972

58. De La Cruz F, Laveck FD: Human Sexuality and the Mentally Retarded. New York, Brunner-Mazel, 1973

59. Birnbaum M: The right to treatment, Am Bar Assoc J, 46:499–503, 1960

60. Rouse v Cameron 373 F.2d 451, D.C. Cir 1966

61. Covington v Harris 419 F.2d 617, D.C. Cir 1969
62. Wyatt v Stickney, Civil No. 3195–N, M.D. Ala. 1972
63. The President's Committee on Mental Retardation, Annual Report, Washington, DC, 1969
64. Murdock: op cit, p 171
65. Schultz T: The handicapped, a minority demanding its rights, New York Times, February 13, 1977, p E8
66. Roe v Wade 410 U.S. 113, 1973
67. Grad FP: Public Health Law Manual. New York, Am Public Health Assoc 1970, p 5
68. Swazey J: Phenylketonuria: a case study in biomedical legislation. J Urban Law 483, 1971, p 833
69. Reilly PR: Sickle cell anemia legislation. J Leg Med, 1973, p 39
70. Reilly PR: The role of law in the prevention of genetic disease. In Milunsky A: op cit, pp 428–29. See also Murry RF: Problems behind the promise: ethical issues in mass-genetic screening. Hastings Cent Rep, April 1972, pp 10–13
71. Ibid., pp 436–37
72. Milunsky A: Genetic counseling: principles and practice. In Milunsky A: op cit, pp 64–65
73. World Health Organization Expert Committee: Genetic Counseling. WHO Tech Rep 416:1, 1969
74. Sorenson JR: Counselors: self portrait. Genetic Counseling 1, 1973, p 31
75. Capron AM: Informed decision-making in genetic counseling. Indiana Law J 48:581, 1973
76. Downie RS, Telfer E: Respect for Persons. New York, Schocken Books, 1970, p 93. See also Fletcher JF: Four indicators of humanhood. Hastings Cent Rep, December 1974, pp 4–7
77. Kant I: The Fundamental Principles of the Metaphysic of Morals. Translated by Paton HJ: The Moral Law. London, Hutchinson's University Library, 1948, pp 90–91
78. Downie RS, Telfer E: op cit, p 19
79. Ramsey P: Fabricated Man: The Ethics of Genetic Control. New Haven, Yale University Press, 1970
80. Rorvik DM: Making men and women without men and women. Esquire, April 1969, pp 108–15
81. Bronowski J: Science and Human Values. New York, Harper, 1956
82. Lappé M: Can eugenic policy be just? In Milunsky A: op cit, pp 456–58
83. Guttman F: On withholding treatment: Can Med Assoc J 111:520–523, 1974
84. Crocker AC, Cushna B: Ethical considerations and attitudes in the field of developmental disorders. In Johnston RB, Magrab PR: Developmental Disorders: Assessment, Treatment, Education. Baltimore, University Park Press, 1976, p 499
85. Ibid., p 496

86. Donovan P: Sterilizing the poor and the incompetent. Hastings Cent Rep, October 1976, pp 7–8

87. Friedman PR: The Rights of Mentally Retarded Persons. New York, Avon, 1976, pp 115–21

88. Krugman S, Giles JP: Viral hepatitis: new light on an old disease. JAMA 212:1019–21, 1970

89. Goldby S: Letter. Lancet, April 10, 1971, p 749

90. Krugman S: Letter. Lancet, May 8, 1971, p 966

91. Edsall G: Letter. Lancet, July 10, 1971, p 95

92. Ramsey P: The Patient as Person. New Haven, Yale University Press, 1970, pp 40–58

93. Gibson BS, Reed JC: Training nurses in mental retardation. Ment Retard 12(6):19–22

94. Smiley CW: Sterilization and therapeutic abortion counseling for the mentally retarded. J Psych Nurs, May–June 1974, pp 24–26

95. Mahoney JA: Viewpoints on attitudes and actions towards handicapped children. J Pract Nurs, April 1974, pp 40–41

96. Symposium on the child with developmental disabilities. Nurs Clin North Am, June 1975

97. Haynes M: Teaching mental retardation nursing. Am J Nurs, April 1975, pp 626–28

98. Hume PJ: Perspectives in nursing the mentally handicapped. World IR Nurs, June 1975, pp 6–7

99. Branson HK: The nurse's role in behavior modification. Nurs Care, December 1975, pp 21–23

100. Thurman RL, et al: The nurse practitioner and institutional facilities for the mentally retarded—are they compatible? J Psych Nurs, May, 1976, pp 7–10

101. Horoshak I: Where hope for mentally retardees grows brighter—Eunice Kennedy Shriver Center for Mental Retardation. RN, June 1976, pp 39–43

102. Hannam C: Parents and Mentally Handicapped Children. Baltimore, Penguin Books, 1975, p 48

103. Mageroff M: On Caring. New York, Harper & Row, 1971

10

PUBLIC POLICY AND HEALTH CARE DELIVERY

INTRODUCTION

Public policy consists of the principles guiding action of society as a whole.[1] These principles are or should be the concern of everyone in that society. Issues of public health policy and ethics intersect in considerations of just distribution of health and nursing care to individuals and groups at local, state, national, and international levels. Nurses are involved in recommending and making policy from institutional to international levels of governance. Examples of this involvement range on a continuum from setting fiscal policies that determine who will get nursing care in a given area to the more dramatic decisions about whether or not recombinant DNA research should be carried on in a particular community.[2]

All health policy issues involve value dimensions that are often not considered in the heat of debate over economic and political factors. Economist E.F. Schumacher warns that economic judgments are fragmentary, usually short term, and that other values need to be considered.[3] The *1976 Report on National Growth and Development* also says that the economic system alone cannot meet all the social needs of the nation.[4] Arguments and decisions about policy are ultimately based on underlying assumptions about what is valued in society and where health is placed on the scale of competing social values. In listing major grievances, most Americans today still place drugs, crime, high cost-of-living, inflation, housing, schools, unemployment, and corruption in government above health care.[5] This is significant to nurses as providers and consumers of health and nursing care for it means that finite resources must be allocated among competing interests such as education, housing, and welfare, broadly and more narrowly within the field of health itself. Curative and preventive care and teaching and research represent competing interests and claims. No one knows quite how to deal with the fact that 67 percent of our total national health expenditures in 1975 was on hospital expenses, physician services, and on drug costs, a total of $80 billion. Total health expenditures for that year amounted to $119 billion or 8.3 percent of the gross national product.[6]

Fuchs, another economist, points out that resources are scarce, resources have alternative uses, and people have different wants and attach different levels of importance to satisfying these wants.[7] Notice that Fuchs is talking about wants, not needs. Needs, to philosophers Frankena and Rawls, could be used as one basis for distribution of benefits and burdens in a just fashion, health care, for example. The three factors, mentioned by Fuchs, make choices imperative at personal and social levels. What is the most just and fair distribution? Who is to choose beyond the personal level for a community or a nation? Who should decide where resources will go and what human "wants" will be acknowledged and met? How will priorities be set? How will the needs of the individual and of society be reconciled? How much weight do we want to give to equality and individual freedom of choice? How important is health? Is there a "right" to health? These and numerous other questions raise issues that reflect the basic values of our pluralistic society.

The Brookings Institution in Washington, D.C. publishes documents periodically with the purpose of assisting in development of sound public policy and promoting public understanding of nationally important policy issues. One such document, *Setting National Priorities,* sets out the proposed federal budget, stating executive branch decisions about national priorities. In it, one sees the role of the federal government as the "equalizer of resources" among citizens and among state and local governments.[8] The chapter on health care dealt primarily with medical care cost inflation and the appropriate role of the federal government in providing health insurance and designing a mechanism to carry it out in the face of conflicting objectives of providers, consumers, government, and insurance companies. The author also points out that medical care is only one factor contributing to health.[9] Medical care does not equal health.[10,11]

Efforts "to promote the general welfare" represent part of the overall purpose of government as found in the Preamble to the U.S. Constitution. Public policy develops within the constitutional framework to meet this goal. According to Strickland the policy-making process consists of deciding on goals for the public good, and delineating and activating strategies for achieving these goals. This process requires agreement on both means and ends among those who have effective control over resources such as money, manpower, and facilities.[12] One is hard put to find a national health policy per se if one considers the four aspects essential to policy: clear statement of purpose, working consensus to achieve the purpose, agreement on both means and ends and continuing, and focused fiscal support of composite programs.[13] At the present time most American medical care is focused primarily on disease care; we talk prevention, yet most insurance provides coverage for hospital care and physicians' services in the hospital. Relatively few people have insurance coverage for preventive or ambulatory care.[14]

It has been said that we do not have a national health policy per se in the United States. But the federal budget of the executive branch and health legislation for authorizing particular appropriations reflect values and a framework for policy in allocation of hospital beds, medical resources, health manpower, and personal health services at primary, secondary, and tertiary levels.

HISTORICAL AND LEGISLATIVE BACKGROUND

Health and health care seem to have moved into an increasingly prominent place on the national public policy agenda as a social issue. In 1969, HEW issued *Toward a Social Report* identifying health and illness as a major area of social concern.[15] Yet one looks at the *1976 Report on National Growth and Development: The Changing Issues for National Growth* and does not find health care identified in "some of the most important problems and opportunities facing the nation."[16] This may be a reflection of the competing areas of social concern at the federal level. However, government's changing commitment to health as an item on the public policy agenda can be traced historically in legislation and funds actually appropriated to implement the legislation. Hints of a national health policy can be identified from the days of the Colonies.

Early health measures passed by the Colonies in the late 1600s had to do with quarantine for communicable disease control. Further quarantine laws were passed by individual states to control yellow fever. In the 1790s the actual occurrence and continuing threat of yellow fever and its effect on the economy forced the new Congress to pass legislation giving the President power to state the conditions of quarantine. At the time, the debate focused primarily on state versus federal authority rather than health matters per se. In 1813, Congress went further in committing the federal government to more involvement with preservation of health of citizens; a vaccination law was passed to make effective cowpox vaccine available to anyone requesting it free of charge. This law was repealed after the wrong vaccine was sent to the state of North Carolina with disastrous results. (Similar problems still seem to exist in the 1970s with legislation of vaccine programs for all citizens, e.g., swine flu vaccine.[17]) However, a precedent had been set for involvement of the federal government in the health of individual citizens.[18]

In the late 1800s the AMA made a definite distinction between public health and private individual health. "State medicine" was to benefit communities by dealing with diseases that were not strictly limited to individuals and could only be controlled through public efforts, e.g., smallpox. Even at that time, though, there were problems in this distinction that were rapidly blurred. These years saw the beginning of conflict between private groups, primarily the AMA, and government over governmental involvement in health. Another yellow fever epidemic in the 1870s influenced the authorization of a National Board by the federal government. The Board's duties were rather vague. But in the four years of its existence, it did authorize funds for biomedical research.[19]

Problems continued with the quarantine law. Eventually authority was given to the Marine Hospital Service which became the United States Public Health Service in 1912. The Public Health Service was authorized to do epidemiological research in order to control and prevent disease. Preventive medicine and the health of the public was still the general philosophy for government in health matters. Curative medicine and the health of individuals were still primarily private concerns.[20]

European social- and health-insurance schemes began to receive attention in the United States in the early 1900s. The climate of economic reform in the U.S., demands for better working conditions, emergence of labor unions, and passage of the National Health Insurance Act in Britain (1911) stimulated this interest. In the U.S., the American Section of the International Association for Labor Legislation promoted the health-insurance cause by calling for insurance against accidents, sickness, old age, and unemployment. Government recognition of social and health needs was reflected in presidential messages beginning with Theodore Roosevelt in the twentieth century. Federally sponsored health insurance was at least mentioned in many of the presidential messages, but was not activated through legislation. At this time, the AMA was not in opposition to some form of health insurance. This lack of opposition soon ended.[21]

The Great Depression and the passage of the Social Security Act in 1935 saw further federal concern over health even though the Social Security Board had no charge directly related to health insurance when the Act was passed in its final form. In 1939, Senator Robert F. Wagner introduced an amendment to the social security law called the National Health Act of 1939. This was followed in the early 1940s by several attempts to pass the Murray-Wagner-Dingell Bill, which would have created a system of federal compulsory health insurance and federal support of medical education. This proposal never came to a vote. It was strongly opposed by the private side of medical care, the AMA. However, the AMA did support the Hill-Burton Bill (1946), which provided grants-in-aid to hospitals via the states for hospital construction. This program has been steadily extended through the years in the form of grants for such areas as research on hospital utilization, construction of nursing homes and other facilities, and for hospital modernization projects.[22] This was part of an overall effort to improve services to citizens. Actually, this legislation demonstrates the philosophy of sick care in public policy-making, not health care.

Legislative forerunners to Medicare began to appear in the late 1950s and early 1960s in the Forand Bill and the Kerr-Mills Bill, which became law in 1960. The Forand Bill provided hospital and medical care for the elderly through Social Security. Kerr-Mills did not use the Social Security mechanism for financing, but provided federal aid to the states for payments for medical care of "medically indigent" elderly.[23] Before Medicare and Medicaid (Social Security Amendments of 1965) were finally passed, the AMA did introduce its own proposal, Eldercare, which also excluded the Social Security financing mechanism.

Medicare (Title XVIII) and Medicaid (Title XIX) are financing mechanisms and make no provisions for change in the structure of health care delivery. Medicare provides health insurance for the aged (65 and over) and has two parts. Part A provides benefits for hospital inpatient services and posthospital home health services with stipulated periods of time for which benefits are provided. Part B is supplementary medical insurance for such benefits as physicians' services, diagnostic procedures, home health services, outpatient physical therapy, and speech pathology services. The individual must pay a monthly premium for Part B, which is matched by the government. Part B payments may be picked up by Medicaid for the medically indigent aged.[24]

Medicaid provides grants to states for medical assistance programs. Matching federal grants are made available to the states, at state option, for a medical assistance program for such groups as recipients of federally aided public assistance, recipients of supplemental security income benefits, medically indigent in comparable groups (families with dependent children as defined for public assistance purposes, the aged, blind and disabled), and other indigent children. Services are to include inhospital services, outpatient hospital services, other laboratory and x-ray services, skilled nursing home services, physicians' services, screening programs for children and family planning services. Medicaid is usually administered through the Department of Public Welfare or Social Services at the discretion of the individual states.[25] There have been many problems in the implementation of Medicaid legislation.

A look at the Social Security Act Titles passed through the past four decades demonstrates increasing involvement of the federal government in efforts to make health and medical care benefits available to an ever-increasing number of groups, e.g., elderly, disabled, and children. A similar trend can be seen in the Public Health Service Act of 1944, legislating particular activities related to research and investigation of both physical and mental health problems, federal–state cooperation in prevention and control of communicable disease, and medical care to specified groups such as merchant seamen and federal employees. Under this Act, for example, the National Cancer Institute was established, as were Regional Medical Programs (Heart Disease, Cancer and Stroke Amendments of 1965) and Health Manpower legislation (1960), providing grants for training in public health and nursing.[26]

The Comprehensive Health Planning Amendments were passed in 1966. One purpose of this legislation was to encourage comprehensive health planning through establishment of state and areawide comprehensive health planning "A" and "B" agencies. These were primarily review and recommending bodies with a consumer majority, and did not specifically attempt to change the delivery of health care in any major way. The Health Maintenance Organization Act of 1973 provided financial assistance for the development of health maintenance organizations (HMO), which generally include prepaid group practice and Foundations for Medical Care. This was the first deliberate legislative effort at the federal level to reorganize the delivery of health care.[27] In some areas, existing neighborhood health centers were converted into HMOs.

The 1972 Amendments (H.R.1) are particularly interesting as they made important changes in the Social Security Act, including Medicare and Medicaid. These Amendments established Professional Standards Review Organizations (PSROs) directed to problems of control of cost, quality, and medical necessity of services. PSROs are to be established in states for review of professional activities of physicians and other providers, and also institutions that provide services in designated geographical areas. Another provision is for treatment of chronic renal disease under Medicare, with reimbursement provided for hemodialysis and/or renal transplantation in treatment centers for persons insured under Social Security and their dependents.[28]

PL93–641, the National Health Planning and Resource Development Act of 1974, combines many of the activities of Hill-Burton, Regional Medical Programs and Comprehensive Health Planning into one single network of authority with Health Systems Agencies (HSAs) in designated health service areas. Federal funding coming into an area for planning and development of health services will go through these agencies composed of a majority of consumers on the HSA board or executive committee and providers. All must live in the health service area.[29] Some have said that this legislation facilitates having structures in place for implementation of national health insurance.

Appropriation of increasing amounts of funding for medical research and development of the National Institute of Health during the past few decades represents a significant level of governmental support for these activities, even though the amount of funding is now leveling off. At the same time, the National Institute of Health supports its own research efforts and also provides subsidies for medical research in universities and medical schools. These developments assume that medical research was a national priority even though there was no national health policy containing a statement to this effect.

The 1960s and 1970s have seen further development of federal commitment to support of health manpower development. Funding in various forms was appropriated for training of physicians, dentists, pharmacists, nurses, podiatrists, and allied health professionals. Construction grants, improvement grants, student-loan funds, scholarships, and capitation grants were provided to educational and health institutions. The Comprehensive Health Manpower Training Act of 1971 provided for a new program of grants, contracts, and health manpower education initiative awards for the purpose of "improving the distribution, supply, quality, utilization, and efficiency of health personnel and the health services delivery system."[30]

This very brief overview of legislative patterns related to health matters reflects critical choices made over the years in allocation of finite resources from control of communicable disease to development of medical research, health manpower, financing mechanisms for medical and health care, and efforts to alter health care delivery structures. These legislative efforts also underline the fact that money alone has not solved problems of health care delivery.[31] Federal concerns about health of citizens is also reflected in other kinds of legislation not discussed in this chapter, e.g., legislation for regulation of the pharmaceutical industry, vocational rehabilitation, industrial health and safety, the Economic Opportunity Act, and Model Cities.

OTHER INFLUENCES ON HEALTH CARE DELIVERY POLICY

Other factors influencing choices for allocation of resources and health care legislation include consumer unrest and the patients' rights movement. Both consumers and providers are presently involved at the advisory and policy-making levels in health care delivery structures.

Many decisions made today in science and medicine go beyond the scientific and medical arenas into the political and moral. They affect the welfare of scientists and nonscientists alike, e.g., genetic-screening programs and recombinant DNA research. To say that the public is affected by these decisions and supports the technology used in science and medicine does not automatically assume any input into crucial decisions affecting society at large. Although ethical and moral implications of scientific and medical decisions are increasingly recognized, actual priorities can still usually be seen best in terms of proposed budgets and funds appropriated. Society at large should have input into these decisions, e.g., what kinds of biomedical research should be supported and what is the importance of this research when compared with other pressing national priorities. Gaylin says that the public has various mechanisms for influencing the scientific community through legislation, through funding priorities of scientific research agencies, through insistence on education of the public by the scientific community, and by having scientists appear before governmental committees for purposes of articulating problems and serving an educational function for Congress and the public at large.[32]

One example of a cooperative interdisciplinary effort to influence what and how research should be carried on is the National Commission for the Protection of Human Subjects of Biomedical and Behavioral Research, created by Congress in the National Research Act of 1974. The Commission, by law, has a majority of nonresearchers and is mandated to recommend guidelines to the Secretary of HEW for research involving human subjects funded by HEW, to recommend proposals to Congress for regulating non-HEW funded research, and to deliberate whether or not various guidelines developed by the Commission should be extended to federally funded health care delivery efforts. To date this is one of the most extensive efforts to provide for governance of scientific research in the biomedical community at the federal level of policy making.[33]

Health care policy cannot be the monopoly of providers any more than scientists should have the only say on biomedical research. The following reasons are provided as rationale for this position: large amounts of federal funding from taxes for health care, conflicts of interest in the health professions' involvement in controversial activities, many medical decisions have dimensions for which physicians are not specifically trained or have authority, the possibility that these nonmedical dimensions of a health problem (e.g., lifestyle and the environment) may be the critical aspects, health may be valued differently by lay people and by health professionals, and that individual liberty and autonomy extend not only into the political area but also into one's health care. At the present time processes for articulating the voice of consumers in policy-making decisions in health care and research are developing slowly. Municipal as well as voluntary hospitals create community advisory boards; universities and other research institutions develop advisory and review committees to protect human subjects. These are generally interdisciplinary in composition, like the National Commission. Community boards for the municipal hospitals in New York City are expected to participate in establishing planning priorities, allocating funds, judging acceptability of services to clients and areawide planning for delivery of health services.[34]

One of the major problems of lay boards has been access to needed information, e.g., budget plans and on-going research. At times they have resorted to legal action to gain information necessary for decision making or resigned en masse.[35] This problem demonstrates the power of expertise in controlling decisions, and again raises the question as to how patients and community members can effectively influence policy making and policy conflicts in health care. Legislation, education, and cooperation of health care providers are needed in this area as beginning steps to effective consumer participation. The executive boards of HSAs provide another proving ground for the effectiveness of consumer input into policy making.

In April 1976 the Airlie House Conference on Biomedical Research and the Public was convened to discuss more effective ways for Congress and the biomedical research community to communicate with and educate each other. This conference was initiated by Senators Edward M. Kennedy and Jacob K. Javits. The diffuse nature of the problems posed at the conference revealed the need for further dialogue and participants did not come up with specific recommendations. The need for public participation in decision making about scientific research was further reinforced while acknowledging the difficulty of defining the "public." Ideas proposed for further work included the importance of research into finding ways to facilitate public participation in the biomedical research process and health care planning.[36] In the meantime, states and communities are convening their own citizen groups to look at and make recommendations in such areas as recombinant DNA research.[37,38] A public forum on this research for educational purposes was held by the National Academy of Sciences, Washington, D.C., March 1977, another example of the scientific community's attempt to communicate with citizens.

PUBLIC POLICY PROBLEMS IN HEALTH: ETHICAL DIMENSIONS

There are a number of public policy issues in health and related areas that have ethical dimensions, e.g., national health insurance, screening for genetic diseases, and population policies. Renal dialysis, nursing care in the community, medical resources, representation on PSROs, and recombinant DNA research have been selected for discussion purposes.

The issue of finite resource allocation is clearly seen in the provisions of Public Law 92–603 passed in 1972. Patients who require hemodialysis or transplantation for end-stage renal disease are eligible for Medicare, which will pay 80 percent of the costs. This program has proved to be about 50 percent more costly than anticipated. More than 23,000 patients are now enrolled (1976) at a total cost of over 300 million dollars per year. Reimbursement is for treatment in or supervised by kidney disease centers that meet DHEW requirements. Fox says that since dialysis is now financially available to all it has become much more difficult for some renal dialysis teams to justify denying this treatment to any person in renal failure. Yet there is doubt that it is medically, socially, psychologically or financially correct to use this treatment for all cases. If all patients with end-stage renal disease should not be put on dialysis, then someone must look again at criteria for selection. Should the patient's home situation be considered? Should "the will to live" be a major criteria? How can this be determined and by whom should it be?[39,40]

Problems of "quality of life" arise for many patients on dialysis awaiting transplant. Life becomes an endless cycle of treatments, surgery, and rejection of the transplanted kidney, while the patient continues a chronic form of dying. Another question frequently raised is why renal disease is covered financially in this way and other catastrophic diseases are not. The National Kidney Foundation has been very effective as a lobbying group. Do we want to change health care delivery by lobbying for particular diseases? Is this the best way to allocate scarce resources?[41]

Another area that raises the question of who should get care when not all can get care is in the delivery of nursing and health care in the community setting. If specific funding is available for Medicare patients, should more nursing personnel be provided for care of this population group in a nursing agency? If one focuses on this group to the extent that 80–85 percent of an agency case load is composed of persons over 65, then who is providing nursing services to mothers and children and follow-up for discharged patients with psychiatric illness or the mentally retarded, who are returned to the community with inadequate continuity of care plans? Who is responsible for follow-up, the residential institution, community nursing agencies or agencies that do not presently exist? Should care be predicted on ability to pay or some other criteria such as need? In some communities it has been consumer, citizen, and self-help groups that have called attention to the need for follow-up of persons discharged from institutions. If existing agencies cannot provide adequate continuity of care, how will priorities be set? Who should decide? For whom?

Control of recombinant DNA research (a recently developed technique that combines DNA segments from two different organisms) is another policy issue with ethical dimensions. If government is concerned about the welfare of living citizens, what about the welfare of future generations? Should this biologic research—which creates new, potentially dangerous, life forms—be carried on at all? A moratorium on this research was declared in 1975 at the Asilomar Conference in California until guidelines for research in this area could be devised by the National Institutes of Health (NIH) Recombinant DNA Advisory Committee looking at potential biohazards and benefits. These guidelines are applicable to NIH-funded research, but the question remains as to control of the research carried on by private industry and the Defense Department. Walters suggests that along with the immediate issues of hazard and safety there is the long-range question of how we as a society want to actually use new techniques such as the recombinant DNA.[42]

In Cambridge, Massachusetts, the city council's Review Board examined what levels of recombinant DNA research should be allowed at Harvard and MIT. The membership of the Board was a businessman, two nurses, a "community activist," a university professor of urban policy, an engineer, a former city councillor, and a physician specializing in infectious disease.[43] This Review Board represents one way of getting citizen input into controversial questions of health and safety involving the welfare of all citizens in one community.

The establishment of Performance Standard Review Organizations by federal legislation raises the question of who should participate in control of care and cost in hospital care. As biomedical researchers have particular values and interests, so do medical professionals. How can the interests of society be represented in these organizations when it is mandated that only specific providers are to be represented? Page says that the question needs to be raised as to ownership of the professions in a democratic society. Each profession insists on "its" own expertise and autonomy, and seeks to influence public policy decisions affecting the profession. Page, however, claims that the professions belong to society and that society should logically be involved in policy decisions affecting the health and well-being of all.[44] This kind of input from consumers is not required in the PSRO legislation. Should it be mandated? Illich says that as long as doctors alone decide what constitutes good service and assign the sick role they cannot be told what medical services will cost or how many people will be assigned the sick role.[45]

As the Health Service Agencies develop with the mandated majority of consumers on executive boards, the impact of consumer input may be more pronounced. But control of medical services will not be readily shared, as evidenced by AMA activities in the past and the continuing debate over health and medical care as a right. Those who oppose the concept of a right to health care are particularly concerned that rights imply duties. Perhaps if this right does exist, then health professionals, doctors, and nurses are obligated to provide services, a conflict of interest between rights of people to medical and health care and rights of professionals to practice as they please.[46]

Whether medical resources such as blood and organs for transplant purposes should be gifts or commodities is another social problem with ethical dimensions. Using blood as an example, Titmuss, in his book *The Gift Relationship,* compares the voluntary British and the commercial American systems of obtaining blood as to their effectiveness in terms of availability, sufficiency of supply, and wastage. The British system seems to have advantages that the American system does not have in social and economic terms, namely, blood is free in Britain but not in the United States. Questions have been raised about Titmuss' data, but the notion of a gift forces health professionals and society to examine the ethics involved in obtaining those resources used in medical care that can only be contributed by human beings, e.g., blood, organs.[47] Should individuals be required to make certain kinds of donation for the "good" of others?

The above situations and questions provide us with examples of complex social issues with ethical dimensions in the public policy arena. These dilemmas have economic, legal, social, and political ramifications as well. They also demonstrate the interdependence of problem areas in public policy at all levels of governmental concern for health.

ETHICAL DIMENSIONS OF PUBLIC POLICY

The realm of politics is a twilight zone where ethical and technical issues meet.

Reinhold Niebuhr

The literature in the field of public policy and ethics is somewhat limited. One group doing research in this area is the task force on health policy at the Institute for Society, Ethics and the Life Sciences, Hastings Center. Individuals in other organizations, such as the Kennedy Institute, are also looking at this crucial area where ethics and technology intersect.

Social scientists Kelman and Warwick wrote a most significant article for this area of social concern on the ethics of social intervention in the early 1970s. They see social intervention on a continuum from national population policy to policy making in neighborhood action programs and experimentation with human subjects. They see the concept of intervention encompassing broader human endeavors than the concept of "planned change" per se and the ethics of a specific change agent.[48] Social intervention is regarded as any planned or unplanned action that changes characteristics of an individual or the pattern of relationships between individuals.[49] In this chapter, the focus is on the latter concept with attention given to issues in the social and political arenas.

The authors distinguish four aspects of any social intervention that raise major ethical issues[50]: (1) the choice of goals for the proposed change which maximizes certain values and minimizes others, (2) definition of the target of change, i.e., individuals or their environment(s), (3) means chosen to implement the intervention, and (4) evaluation of the consequences of the intervention. For example, if the government contemplates putting a major effort into delivery of preventive health care, this might maximize the value of the greatest good for the greatest number but at the same time might have negative effects on the values of equality and justice for the very sick elderly. In this example, the choice for a target of change might be individual behavior or carcinogenic elements in the environment. Methods of inducing change might impinge on values of individual freedom and autonomy or on freedom of industry to maximize profits. Conflicts might be created between groups working for change in behavior and those working for environmental changes as they compete for scarce resources. Finally, one has to assess the risks and benefits of various consequences of the proposed change on traditional values, e.g., doing all one can for the individual patient. What are we willing or unwilling to give up in the interests of social change? Whose values should prevail?[51]

One key issue in examining goals of intervention and means for implementing change is the extent to which affected population groups have their values and interests represented in the process, e.g., various socioeconomic groups, men, women, children, employed, unemployed, healthy, sick, providers, and consumers. How much control do the affected groups and individuals have in the process of change? Are freedom and self-determination limited by the change process? Whose interests are being served by the proposed intervention, the proposers of a community health program or the target population? Is the power of one group strengthened at the expense of another? All of these concerns should be considered in any process of social intervention. They often are not because of the difficulty in discerning which values should predominate and the difficulty of predicting consequences of particular actions on any selected value, e.g., the freedom of the individual or the welfare of society.[52]

Having mentioned some general difficulties in asking and answering ethical questions in public policy, authors Jonsen, a bioethicist, and Butler, a professor of health policy, suggest some more specific ways that ethical dimensions can be added to policy debate. Dialogue between politicians and ethicists is not commonly carried on in "back rooms" or anywhere else. The concerns of moral philosophy about the "right" and the "good" are not usually considered in developing public policy. In proposing that ethical considerations be part of public policy debate there are several problems considered by these authors that make this dialogue difficult:[53] (1) the fact that ethics does not say which action is right in a given situation, (2) the special language of ethics, (3) the common conception that ethics has to do primarily with personal behavior, (4) the fact that policy makers have constituencies with loyalties and interests that moral philosophers do not, and (5) the fact that policy makers use the technical expertise of others in making decisions but feel that in ethics and moral judgments one is his own expert. Yet both ethicists and policy makers are concerned about what is "good" for society.

Jonsen and Butler see "public ethics" as a subset of social ethics. "Public ethics" deals with public decisions about matters of public concern, e.g., safe and adequate water supply, deals with pressing issues that need decisions, and does not usually expect to create significant structural change in society but involves relatively minor modifications in social or economic arrangements. The three tasks of "public ethics" are (1) to articulate the moral principles most relevant to the policy problem under consideration, e.g., justice, equity, (2) to examine proposed policy choices in view of relevant moral principles, and (3) to rank the order of the moral options for a particular policy choice, i.e., a "moral balance sheet," in terms of which social or economic arrangements will meet one moral principle and not another, e.g., types of health care available in one region and not another.[54] Kelman and Warwick discussed the maximization of certain values and the minimization of others in relation to choice of goals for intervention.

In looking at the development of a national health insurance system, these authors consider two moral principles of distributive justice (fair distribution of harm and benefits in society according to standards of equity, desert, need, or contract) and respect for individuals (implies equal treatment for each person, sets of liberties and rights and obligations). What would the contribution of the ethicist be to debate with lawyers, economists, and physicians about deductibles and co-insurance? This is one example of how a discussion might evolve between a congressman and an ethicist. In bringing the concept of distributive justice into the debate, questions would be raised about the distribution of burdens and benefits to particular groups in society, whether or not equality is a criterion for distribution, the justification of unequal distribution according to merit or ability, and whether there is an "objective" way to determine a "fair" distribution in terms of the most medically needy.[55]

In clarifying policy options, one must, for example, clearly understand the impact of deductibles and co-insurance on the poor, who may be particularly discouraged by them from seeking medical care. If relatively small deductibles are paid by patients, then the money "saved" by government could be used for seriously or chronically ill who must be institutionalized for care. However, wouldn't it be more just to still provide "free" care for the very poor? This might be considered unfair for those who do pay the deductible because there would be less money "saved" to be used for the more expensive care. The ethicist might then show that the criterion of need takes preference over the criterion of equality, the need arising from illness and poverty. In the Rawlsian tradition one might claim that it is not "unfair" to improve the position of the least advantaged in society. In view of fiscal constraints, some rationing of care is necessary so it might be more just to have a plan based on balancing needs of the very sick and very poor. Deductibles would vary with income so that the very poor would pay almost nothing. These considerations would add an ethical dimension to actual health policy debate and decisions. One looks at "equity" factors in various proposals in addition to economic evaluation of cost-benefit analysis, administrative implications, and changes in health care delivery.[56]

The authors discussed above suggest ways of structuring the ethical aspects and arguments in the public policy making process. As the economist Fuchs made very clear, these are significant considerations in choices that have to be made about the allocation of finite resources at all levels of government.

IMPLICATIONS FOR NURSING

The nurse collaborates with members of the health professions and other citizens in promoting community and national efforts to meet the health needs of the public.

ANA Code for Nurses, 1976

Accountability to the client and collaboration with other health professionals for purposes of delivering health care suggests that one of the principles nursing can use in looking at conflict of interests and values in policy making is the needs of patients, families, and communities. This is not an unfamiliar process to nurses in assessment and implementation of nursing care. Should it not be part of the policy-making process in a Health Service Agency? Who will raise this principle to the consciousness of all involved in an executive board meeting? Nurses have been urged to become involved in these organizations. Yet, Novello, Fellow of the American Academy of Nursing and chairperson of the Northwestern Pennsylvania HSA, Health Systems Inc., says that nurses who have become involved since its enactment frequently do not have adequate knowledge about the content of the legislation or the power struggles of various individuals and groups.[57] Is it not a moral responsibility for nurses to be prepared before entering the arena of public policy-making?

Returning to the notion of using needs as a basis for distribution of benefits of health care, they may be placed on a continuum from needs that arise in the person, e.g., serious illness, to needs that arise in the social and physical environment, e.g., clean air and safe streets. All of these needs, as distinct from demands, are related to physical and mental health and must compete with other social interests for scarce resources in the political arena. Nurses should be able to articulate these needs as clearly as possible.

Nursing has been trying to gain entrance into the National Performance Standards Review Council (PSROs). Admission has been denied with the rationale that the law would have to be changed to admit professional groups other than medicine. Yet the legislation mandating the establishment of PSROs talks about review of provider care for hospitalized Medicare and Medicaid patients. Sixty percent of hospital budgets is for nursing service and should be included in the reviewing process. Nursing is also trying to gain membership in the Joint Commission on the Accreditation of Hospitals. Several health professions are attempting to do this with no success because the Commission is reluctant to let more groups into the organization, apparently fearing that it will become too large.[58] These are certainly two groups that confront a host of ethical issues related to health care, whether or not they are ever dealt with at a conscious level.

There are several major decisions that individual nurses and organized nursing must make related to (1) the types of health and health-related organizations and at what level, local, state, national, and/or international they will participate, (2) the type of participation, i.e., observer, observer/participant, active participant, and (3) whether or not they will attempt to place ethical dimensions of health policy issues on the agenda along with the economic and social considerations, e.g., questioning the goals of a proposed family-planning program change and clearly identifying the target of change and underlying assumptions of the proposed change (see Table 3).

One of the ANA priorities for 1974–1976 states that the ANA "will assume a more aggressive role in the development and execution of national health policy."[59] The ANA has also gone on record in a resolution on national health insurance that health is a basic human right and comprehensive health services should be guaranteed to all. There are certainly some real and philosophical problems with this stand.[60] For example, do nurses mean that health, health care, or medical care is a basic human right? What policy implications flow from this stand? What are the values, assumptions, and moral principles underlying each of these positions? Has nursing identified them? Nurses as individuals and organized nursing have been and are involved in the political and policy-making arenas working with consumers and providers of care.[61-67] Schaefer claims that while nursing has goals there is no national plan for action in order to accomplish or influence reform in delivery of health and nursing care.[68]

Nurses can choose to become more knowledgeable about the interaction of

Table 3. NURSING, PUBLIC ETHICS AND POLICY MAKING

| Role | Levels of Organization | | | |
	Local	State	National	Intl
Passive observer	*X△○	X△○	X△○	X△○
Observer/participant	X△○	X△○	X△○	X△○
Active participant	X△○	X△○	X△○	X△○

Ethical Dimension—Questions at All Levels

1. What are proposed changes and goals? Which values are maximized and which minimized, e.g., self-determination, equality?

2. What or who is the target of the proposed change? How much control do affected groups and individuals have over the proposed change?

3. What means are used to implement change, e.g., coercion, bribes, education?

4. What are the consequences for present and future populations?

*Individual nurse = X ; informal groups of nurses = △, organized nursing = ○.

social, economic, ethical, and political aspects in institutional and public policy-decisions. They can seek to influence these decisions personally and/or through professional or community group action. Expertise is one form of power and not to choose is a choice in itself. Making these choices requires a careful look at values and assumptions underlying the talk of nursing and the behavior of nursing and nurses in patient, colleague, and community relationships. For example, what does the claim that the nurse is an advocate of the patient imply in terms of policy making and examining the ethical dimensions of this process? What moral principles are violated in a specific policy proposal, e.g., equality, justice, veracity? This is indeed a difficult and complex task. If an underlying value for the nurse is to please everyone, then that value will be reflected in behavior rather than the value of meeting patients' and society's needs for health care. This poses a tremendous challenge to the institutions that educate nurses and to those nurses in leadership positions. Ethical dimensions of health policy-making could well be articulated by the nursing profession in the public policy-arena.

REFERENCES

1. Preston LE, Post JE: Private Management and Public Policy: The Principle of Public Responsibility. Englewood Cliffs, NJ, Prentice-Hall, 1975, p 11
2. Wade N: Gene-splicing: Cambridge citizens OK research but want more safety. Science 195:268, 1977
3. Schumacher EF: Small is Beautiful. New York, Harper & Row, 1973
4. 1976 Report on National Growth and Development: The Changing Issues for National Growth. Third Biennial Report to the Congress submitted pursuant to Section 703(a) of Title VII, Housing and Urban Development Act of 1970, February 1976, p 144
5. Knowles JH: Introduction. Daedalus 4, Winter 1977, p 4
6. Ibid., p 2
7. Fuchs VR: Who Shall Live? New York, Basic, 1974, p 4
8. Schultze CL, Fried ER, Rivlin AM, Teeters NH: Setting National Priorities: The 1973 Budget. Washington, D.C., The Brookings Institution, 1972
9. Ibid., pp 213–14
10. Wildavsky A: Doing better and feeling worse: the political pathology of health policy. Daedalus, Winter 1977, p 105
11. Illich I: Medical Nemesis: The Expropriation of Health. Toronto, McClelland and Stewart, 1975
12. Strickland SP: Politics, Science, and Dread Disease. Cambridge, Mass, Harvard University, 1972, pp x–xi
13. Ibid., p 255
14. Kristein MM, Arnold CB, Wynder EL: Health economics and preventive care. Science 195:475, 1977
15. Preston, Post: op cit, p 81
16. 1976 Report on National Growth and Development. op cit, p ii
17. Boffey PM: Guillain–Barré: Rare disease paralyzes Swine Flu Campaign. Science 195:155–159, 1977
18. Chapman CB, Talmadge JM: The evolution of the right to health concept in the United States. Pharos 34:31–33, 1971
19. Ibid., p 35
20. Ibid., pp 35–36
21. Ibid., pp 40, 42
22. Stevens R: American Medicine and the Public Interest. New Haven, Yale University, 1971, p 510
23. Wilson FA, Neuhauser D: Health Services in the United States. Cambridge, Mass, Ballinger, 1974, p 124
24. Ibid., pp 143–44
25. Ibid., pp 145–46
26. Ibid., p 161
27. Ibid., pp 166–68

28. Ibid., pp 138-42
29. Novello DJ: The National Health Planning and Resources Development Act. Nurs Outlook 24:354-58, 1976
30. Wilson, Neuhauser: op cit, p 164
31. Wildavsky: op cit, p 105
32. Gaylin W: Scientific research and public regulation. Hastings Cent Rep, June 1975, p 7
33. Steinfels P: The National Commission and fetal research: Introduction. Hastings Cent Rep, June 1975, p 11
34. Veatch L: Community boards in search of authority. Hastings Cent Rep, October 1975, p 28
35. Ibid., p 29
36. Steinfels P: Research and the public: a report from the Airlie House Conference. Hastings Cent Rep, June 1976, pp 21-25
37. Wade: op cit, pp 268-269
38. Wade N: Recombinant DNA: New York State ponders action to control research. Science 194:705-6, 1976
39. Perkoff G et al: Long-term dialysis programs: new selection criteria, new problems—the impact of federal funding. Hastings Cent Rep, June 1976, pp 11-13
40. Fox RC, Swazey JP: The Courage to Fail. Chicago, University of Chicago, 1974, pp 274-79
41. Perkoff et al: op cit, p 12
42. Walters L: Recombinant DNA molecule research: the search for a balance between safety and progress. Kennedy Ins Q Rep, Spring 1976, p 3
43. Wade N: op cit
44. Page BB: Who owns the professions? Hastings Cent Rep, October 1975, pp 7-8
45. Illich: op cit, pp 76-77
46. Jameton AL: Moral problems on a social scale: introduction. In Gorovitz S, Jameston AL, Macklin R, O'Connor JM, Perrin EV, St. Clair BP, Sherwin S (eds): Moral Problems in Medicine. Englewood Cliffs, NJ, Prentice-Hall, 1976, pp 426-28
47. Solow RM: From Blood and Thunder. In Gorovitz S et al (eds): Moral Problems in Medicine. Englewood Cliffs, NJ, Prentice-Hall, 1976, pp 510-21
48. Benne KD: Some ethical problems in group and organizational consultation. In Bennis WG, Benne KD, Chin R (eds): The Planning of Change. New York, Holt, Rinehart and Winston, 1961, pp 595-604
49. Warwick DP, Kelman HC: Ethical issues in social intervention. In Zaltman G (ed): Process and Phenomena of Social Change. New York, Wiley, 1973, p 377
50. Ibid., pp 377-79
51. Ibid., pp 379-80
52. Ibid., pp 388-400

53. Jonsen AR, Butler LH: Public ethics and policy making. Hastings Cent Rep, August 1975, pp 20–21
54. Ibid., p 23–24
55. Ibid., p 28
56. Ibid., pp 28–29
57. Novello: op cit, p 354
58. ANA denied membership on JCAH Council. Am Nurs, January 15, 1977, pp 1, 5
59. American Nurses' Association position on National Health Insurance. Am J Nurs 74:1262–63, 1974
60. Callahan D: Health and society: Some ethical imperatives. Daedalus, Winter 1977, pp 30–31
61. Novello: op cit, pp 354–58
62. Paulson VW, Ostberg AJ, Cain ER: Commitment to change in Colorado. Am J Nurs 75:636–37, 1975
63. Nurses urged to heed proliferating "federal regs." Am J Nurs 76:884–88, 889, 1976
64. Zimmerman A: Health Care: Why bypass the nurses? Am Nurs, January 15, 1977, p 5
65. Anne Keith - general award. Mass Nurs 46:5, 1977
66. Milio N: The Care of Health in Communities: Access for Outcasts. New York, MacMillan, 1975, pp 219–98
67. Dock L: Lavinia L. Dock: Self-portrait. Nurs Outlook 25:24–25, 1977
68. Schaefer MJ: Toward a full profession of nursing: the challenge of the educator's role. J Nurs Educ, November 1972, p 40

11

SELECTED
EXAMPLES OF
ETHICAL DILEMMAS

Good decision-making . . . seems to require human sensitivity, illuminating and useful principles, access to pertinent information, methods of weighting and balancing options—reason and feeling, private meditation and public discussion, good sense and good sensibilities.[1]

This chapter presents hypothetical case studies involving ethical dilemmas for the nurse and other health workers. There are two case studies for each of Chapters 4 through 10. Each of the related chapters contains content helpful for consideration of the basic elements of decision making in ethical dilemmas discussed below and for exploration of additional suggested questions that follow each case study. The reader may wish to review Chapter 2 before working with the case studies. In each of these situations, the individual and/or group is seeking the best solution for a given situation where there is, for example, a conflict of duties and rights, a line is or needs to be drawn, or a moral principle is or has been violated.

In order to think systematically about the ethical dilemmas in the case studies, one should consider some basic elements. The first element to be considered is the available data base. The data base may not be as complete as one wishes or considers necessary. However, this is a reality of many decision-making situations. To say that there is a lack of data may be used as a cop-out to impede further discussion, to stall the decision-making process, or to refuse to participate in the critical thinking processes required by ethical dilemmas. The following questions are another element of the decision making process, to be explored as they are appropriate to a given situation:

1. Who should be involved in the decision-making process? Who should make the final decision? Why?
2. For whom should the decision be made, for example, self, proxy, other?
3. What criteria should be used, for example, physiologic condition, economic considerations, psychologic status, legal considerations, social and family considerations?
4. What degree of consent should be obtained from the patient/client?
5. What, if any, moral principles are enhanced or negated by proposed decisions for action, for example, truth-telling, justice, self-determination, respect for the individual?

When thinking about the moral principles involved, one should consider Rawls' criteria of universality, generality, publicity, ordering, and finality. (See Chapter 2 for details of these criteria.)

Underlying efforts to seek the right-making characteristics of actions and solutions to the ethical dilemmas presented, and to determine value, is the third element to be considered. This element is concerned with the various modes of moral reasoning that are involved consciously or subconsciously in the decision-making process. They should be articulated as part of the process as they may result in different decisional outcomes, for example:

1. The utilitarian approach that seeks the greatest good for the greatest number and focuses primarily on consequences of action—frequently used in justifying decisions made in the health care delivery system.
2. The formalist or deontological approach that considers more than just the consequences of an action or rule, for example, the use of moral principles and rules such as respect for the individual and truth telling.
3. The Rawlsian approach that no one should benefit unless all benefit by a proposed action.
4. The approach of a theory of obligation, such as that of Frankena which derives from concepts of beneficence and justice as equal treatment.

Any one of these underlying ways of thinking about ethical dilemmas may come into direct conflict in a given situation with the medical ethic that says that one should do no harm and one should do all that one can for the individual patient.

Articulation of a position on a given ethical issue or in a specific situation of conflict whether at the health worker/client level of interaction or at the policy making level involves thoughtful, sensitive consideration of all the elements mentioned: the available data base, general questions involved in the decision-making process itself, and articulation of the underlying moral and value positions or approaches. The reader may think of additional dimensions that should enter into the equation for decision making about ethical dilemmas. Dilemmas are not resolved immediately through this process, but one gains increased sensitivity to the issues and complexities involved in ethical dilemmas through debate and discussion.

CHAPTER 4: PATIENTS' RIGHTS AND OBLIGATIONS

Case Study 1

Linda and Bob are both 21 years old. They were married right after finishing high school. Bob works at a local gas station as a mechanic. Linda was a waitress and occasionally works now as a cocktail waitress to augment the family income. Both Linda and Bob attend a local community college sporadically. They live in the large second floor apartment of a house owned by Bob's parents who both work at the local steel plant. Linda and Bob have a 20 month-old son and a 5-month-old daughter, both born prematurely.

Linda made attempts to use the pill as a means of birth control as "I'm not too keen on kids." Bob is very much opposed to any form of birth control and this has been the source of many arguments between them. He is Catholic and she was brought up as a Methodist.

The public health nurse (PHN) knows the family through their contacts with the neighborhood health center and has made follow-up home visits after the birth of each child. The PHN has been spending a great deal of time with this family after the birth of the second child due to Linda's hostility and apparent inability to cope with another child. Linda did not want the PHN to come for visits, but finally relented when the hospital said these visits were required in order for the baby to go home. During the last visit, Linda commented to the nurse that, though she did not want anyone to know, she thought that

Bob hurt Billy, the son, when she was working. Billy had bruises on his fore-head and thighs. Bob said that Billy fell off his rocking horse. Linda also mentioned that Bob did not seem very "happy" lately and was recently involved in a fist-fight at a local bar.

The PHN knows vaguely that there is a state law about reporting suspected child abuse. Then she thinks about the progress that she has been making with Linda and the baby daughter. She also recalls that Linda said no one is to know about her suspicions of Bob.

Additional Questions for Discussion

What are the obligations of the PHN in this situation to the children, the parents, the agency, the community, and to herself?

Whose "rights" should take priority? Why?

Should the "right to health care" include nursing service at home?

Case Study 2

John is an "average" high-school student on renal dialysis at home. He is 16 years old and started dialysis for the second time after his kidney transplant began to fail. His kidney problems began after a sports injury a few years ago. He is the second oldest of four children. His older sister is in college and two younger brothers are at home. His mother died two years ago in an auto accident. John's grandmother, a widow, lives with the family now and is the person responsible for helping him with his dialysis at home. John has a close relationship with both his father and grandmother. He has remained generally optimistic until his transplanted kidney began to fail.

On his last visit to the Dialysis Center for a periodic check-up, he confided several things to one of the nurses he has known throughout his illness. He claims he does not want anyone else to know about these things, "I mean it—don't tell anybody, the docs, my dad or my grandmother—nobody." John is thinking about committing suicide. He has not decided how and wonders if the nurse could do something to help or "maybe I just won't have any more of these treatments." He tells the nurse the reason he wants to commit suicide is because he knows his dad is having some business problems and may have trouble paying his sister's college tuition. His younger brother needs some orthodontic work. He also knows that his Dad plans to remarry and his grandmother will probably leave to live in an apartment. He feels that he will probably die soon. "Why drag it out?" On the other hand, he just heard about some new research that Dr. S is doing and maybe he should stay around to participate in it even if it "won't help me."

Additional Questions for Discussion

What are the nurse's obligations to John, his family, the physician, and others involved in his care?

What are John's "rights" to confidentiality?

Should the allocation of family, hospital, and community resources be considered?

Should a teeneager be allowed to refuse treatment? Why, or why not?

Does one have a "right to die"?

CHAPTER 5: INFORMED CONSENT

Case Study 1

Mr. S and his wife have been visiting their 10 year old daughter, Tina, daily since she was admitted to the hospital four days ago. She has a diagnosis of cancer of the liver, but the parents who are on welfare have not been told the diagnosis. The physician feels that the parents, who are Spanish speaking, will not comprehend any of the terminology necessary to understand the diagnosis. The nurses on the unit have described the parents as "dull," but feel that they should have an explanation of Tina's illness in order to give the required informed consent for various procedures. Both Mr. and Mrs. S have asked the nurses about what is going to happen to Tina. They know that Tina is critically ill.

Additional Questions for Discussion

What are the elements of "informed consent"?

What is the nurse's obligation to the parents and to the child to obtain "informed consent"?

How should children participate in the informed consent process?

Case Study 2

Mrs. R is a woman in her mid-40s with multiple sclerosis. She has two teenage daughters, 14 and 16 years old, living at home. Mr. R, a middle-management executive in a local firm, left the home five years ago. Mrs. R often comes into the emergency room of the local community hospital for treatment of acute episodes of asthma. The physician has ordered that if Mrs. R arrests during an acute episode, no CODE should be called. As far as the nurses know, the physician made this decision on his own with no input from the patient or others significant to her or depending on her. One nurse is terribly upset because this decision conflicts strongly with her own professional and personal moral values. She herself has said on several occasions that Mrs. R's home situation is "intolerable" and "I certainly wouldn't want to live under those circumstances." None of the nurses have heard Mrs. R express any similar feelings about her situation even though she usually seems somewhat depressed when she comes into the emergency room.

Additional Questions for Discussion

Does Mrs. R have rights to "informed consent" in this situation?

What, if anything, should the nurse do before Mrs. R comes into the emergency room again?

Does the nurse have an obligation to intervene rather than just "praying" that Mrs. R "doesn't come in on my shift"?

CHAPTER 6: ABORTION

Case Study 1

Joan is an 18-year-old pregnant teenager who is receiving prenatal care at a local neighborhood health center. She had a baby last year that she decided to keep with help from her family with whom she lives. Joan's father is a general practitioner. She has been attending high school and hoped to graduate next year. However, she dropped out of school recently as she had not been feeling "up to par" with this pregnancy. She works part-time as a cashier at one of the local supermarkets.

You are the nurse practitioner caring for Joan, who told you on her first visit that she had been exposed to rubella 3 weeks ago when her little brother and several of his classmates had "the measles." She is just entering the second trimester. You have explained to Joan and her mother the risks to the fetus from this exposure. Her mother wants her to have an abortion, but Joan refuses to have it done, claiming a "right" to have her own child. She and her fiance are deciding whether they should marry or not before the baby is born.

Additional Questions for Discussion

Does one have a "right" to bear children? How many?

Should the nurse practitioner use coercion in this situation to force an individual to have an abortion? Why or why not?

If Joan decides to have an abortion, under what conditions could the fetus be used for research?

Should the unmarried father have any rights in the decision for or against an abortion?

If this child is born with severe deformities, who should pay for its care?

Case Study 2

Mrs. A is a 39-year-old woman, pregnant for the first time. Both she and her husband are Jewish. She was married last year for the second time.

Her physician suggested that she should have an amniocentesis due to the increased risk of Down's syndrome with increased maternal age, as well as the risk of Tay-Sachs disease. Mrs. A was somewhat reluctant because she and her husband are very excited about this pregnancy as it will be the first grandchild in each of their families.

Mrs. A has amniocentesis performed, which shows that the fetus, a female, does have Tay-Sachs disease. The A's are heart broken about the situation and are trying to decide whether or not Mrs. A should have an abortion so that she can become pregnant again as soon as possible.

You are the community health nurse visiting Mrs. A's mother who lives with her daughter and has had a "mild" C.V.A. Mrs. A has been discussing her indecision about the abortion with you.

Additional Questions for Discussion

What are the obligations of the nurse who feels that Mrs. A should definitely have the abortion?

What are the professional health worker's obligations to his or her own personal values in patient interaction?

Does this fetus have a "right" to be born?

What if the A's wanted to abort this fetus simply because they would rather have a boy?

CHAPTER 7: DYING AND DEATH

Case Study 1

Mr. C, a 48-year-old salesman, arrives on your unit with a "living will" to which he has given much thought and attention. He is divorced and remarried and has two children from his second marriage, 9 and 11 years old. Mr. C is having a second surgical procedure for cancer of the bowel after surgery and radiation therapy six months ago. He has been told that he has metastasis to the liver and that he should get his affairs in order.

Living wills are not legally binding in your state and you wonder what to do beyond attaching the will to Mr. C's chart and making sure that everyone caring for Mr. C is aware of this. You do not agree with some of the conditions in Mr. C's living will as stated and wonder if you should try to change his mind. You feel that "extraordinary means" should be used because of Mr. C's children, "they should have their father with them as long as possible." Mr. C's wife has already told you that she thinks a "living will" is totally unnecessary as the "doctors should decide."

Additional Questions for Discussion

How does one distinguish between "ordinary" and "extraordinary" treatment measures in general and for a particular patient?

What does it mean to "die with dignity"?

Should nurses participate in passive or active euthanasia procedures? How? Why, or why not?

Should nurses support legislative efforts to make "living wills" legal? Why or why not?

Case Study 2

Jack is 14 years old. He was brought into the intensive care unit of the local community hospital after an accident while playing football. He has been in a coma and on a respirator since the accident two months ago. Jack's father is manager of a local discount store. His mother is active in church and busy with five other children, all younger than Jack. The youngest has Downs' syndrome and attends a special class at the local public school. The nurses know that Jack's hospitalization is a terrible drain on this family financially and emotionally.

Jack's mother has asked one of the night nurses to "just unplug the respirator sometime when you're on duty. Who's to know?" Jack meets the Harvard brain death criteria. The legislature in Jack's state has recently authorized this criteria as a "legally" acceptable basis for "pulling the plug." The physician has not discussed this with Jack's parents and has adopted a "wait and see" attitude because he knows of a similar case where a patient on a respirator for eight months is now back in school.

Additional Questions for Discussion

Does the nurse have an obligation to bring the mother's request to the physician's attention? Why?

Do Jack's siblings and parents have any "rights" that should be considered in the situation?

What are the nurse's "rights"?

Do nurses have rights, or just duties and obligations?

Whose rights should take priority?

Who should pay for Jack's care now that he is "legally" dead?

CHAPTER 8: BEHAVIOR CONTROL

Case Study 1

Mrs. T is a 42-year-old woman with a history of occasional depressive episodes. Her husband is a successful businessman in their local community. Their third and youngest child is a college freshman in another state. The older children are married. Mrs. T has her own real-estate business that is moderately successful.

Mrs. T is a patient in a private psychiatric facility for a third depressive episode in the past four years. She has been on various medications, but now her psychiatrist has ordered that she have a series of electric shock treatments (EST). Mrs. T refuses these treatments and says that there must be something other than EST that the doctor can prescribe.

Additional Questions for Discussion

What are Mrs. T's "rights" in this situation?

What are the nurse's rights and obligations?

Should Mrs. T's husband be involved in the decision making that occurs? Why?

Can a patient refuse treatment?

Should Mrs. T be forced to have these treatments "for her own good"?

Case Study 2

Bob is an eight-year-old third-grader who has been diagnosed as "hyperactive" by his family doctor, and put on amphetamines so that he can "quiet down and learn something in school." You are the school nurse and are concerned that Bob has not had a complete psychologic or neurologic work-up before he started taking the amphetamines his teacher mentioned to you. You know that Bob's family has had several crisis situations recently, for example, the birth of a new baby and a great-grandfather moving into the home. You feel this makes a complete evaluation for Bob even more critical. You also know that treatment with amphetamines as well as labeling a child "hyperactive" is controversial.

Bob has been an only child until this time and has been described as an average student with "some occasional difficulty in concentrating on his work." Bob's parents both teach school and are very concerned about their son and his academic progress.

Additional Questions for Discussion

What "rights" do children have to health care?

What are some of the problems in assuring that a child's rights are exercised in the health care system?

Should children have rights that adults do not have? If so, what are they?

Do schools have moral, in addition to legal, obligations to make sure that students receive adequate health care?

Should children be given such labels as "hyperactive" or "emotionally disturbed"? Why or why not? What are the risks of such labeling?

CHAPTER 9: MENTAL RETARDATION

Case Study 1

Jane is 19 years old and lives at home with her parents and two "normal" siblings, a brother 16 years old and a sister 9 years old. The father works in a local factory as a foreman. Her mother is at home and cares for Jane's widowed grandmother who recently moved into the home after surgery for an arthritic hip. Jane has Downs' syndrome and is mildly retarded. She goes to a sheltered workshop every day by herself on the bus. She had one out-of-wedlock baby last year, which her parents adopted. They want her to be sterilized, but Jane does not want this done. She insists that she wants to use the pill she gets from her family doctor. She has heard too many horror stories about the IUD from other women at the sheltered workshop.

The only contact that the PHN has had recently with Jane is at the bus stop where Jane waits for the local bus. Yesterday Jane mentioned that she has been robbed twice on her way home from the bus stop and that she thinks she might be pregnant. This has not been confirmed and the nurse refrains from asking her if she has thought about an abortion this time, but does suggest that Jane see her family doctor or go to the neighborhood health center.

Additional Questions for Discussion

Should the nurse intervene any further? How?

Whose rights should be considered in this situation? For example, Jane's rights, her family's rights, etc.?

Should the developmentally disabled be "allowed" to reproduce?

What are the community's obligations to the developmentally disabled?

Should the nurse encourage Jane to have an abortion if they have further conversations?

Does a child have a "right" to "normal" parents?

Case Study 2

The J family is a family of moderate means with five children. Mr. J is a long-distance truck driver. Tommy, the youngest child, age 6, has Downs' syndrome with moderate retardation and lives in a residential school. He was recently hospitalized for surgery.

Mrs. J tells the nurses on the surgical unit that she and her husband have had some pressure from the social worker and other staff of the state residential school to take Tommy back into their home under the policy of deinstitutionalization. Mr. and Mrs. J find the present arrangement satisfactory as Mrs. J also works. They feel that it would be too much of a strain to have Tommy at home again. He was at home for the first year of his life and still needs much supervision. There are community resources available for children of school age, but Mrs. J would have the major responsibility of Tommy's care at home.

One of the nurses said that she would not want Tommy at home. Another said that she felt that Mr. and Mrs. J should take him home, "after all, he is their child and he's not as retarded as some others I've seen."

Additional Questions for Discussion

What are the nurses' obligations to Tommy, to his parents, and to the community?

Should the nurses try to impose different values on Mr. and Mrs. J when their values differ from those of institutional policy?

Should families be coerced into caring for the developmentally disabled at home? If yes, what is the community's obligation to such families?

CHAPTER 10: PUBLIC POLICY AND HEALTH CARE DELIVERY

Case Study 1

The nursing director of a community nursing agency has received notice that certain families in the agency caseload are no longer eligible for Medicaid funds. These funds have been cut back by authorization of the state. The director has also heard recently that the agency will lose two staff nurse positions as well. Agency funds set aside for emergency purposes are exhausted.

All the Medicaid families need continued nursing supervision. The director is also very concerned about the "quality" of nursing care that the nurses can provide in terms of numbers of available staff and the many Medicare patients who continue to increase the agency caseload. New referrals for patients on Medicare arrive daily in the agency.

Additional Questions for Discussion

What are the director's moral obligations to the community, to patients, to the staff, and to the agency?

What "rights" are in conflict?

Should nursing care in the community outside the hospital setting depend on ability to pay?

Do the director of the agency and the agency nurses have the "right" to deliver comprehensive nursing care to anyone needing care?

Should nursing agencies call themselves community nursing agencies if they can only deliver care to one population group, for example, the elderly? Why or why not?

Is the public morally obligated to provide nursing care for everyone needing such care? Why or why not?

Case Study 2

You practice nursing in a state reconsidering its genetic-screening legislation. A group of nurses at the state-wide level has decided to organize and present a position paper to the legislative committee working on genetic screening. Legislation in your state mandates screening for PKU and ten other genetic disorders. You know that many of the conditions screened for presently have no treatment, that parents do not usually give informed consent for this procedure on a hospital newborn unit, and that no provision is made for follow-up. You decide to join the state-wide group to influence changes in the legislation.

Additional Questions for Discussion

What moral principles might be considered in looking at proposed changes in this legislation?

Should informed consent from a parent or both parents be required for genetic-screening procedures? Some, or all?

Whose rights are violated in the present legislation?

What public values are expressed in the present legislation? Do these values conflict with any values that might be held privately by individuals, families, or health professionals?

REFERENCE

1. Callahan D: Values, facts and decision-making. Hastings Cent Rep, June 1971, p 1

AUTHOR INDEX

SUBJECT INDEX